Also by Michael F. Roizen, M.D., and Mehmet C. Oz, M.D.

You: The Owner's Manual

Also by Michael F. Roizen, M.D.

The RealAge Workout: Maximum Health, Minimum Work

The RealAge Makeover: Take Years off Your Looks
and Add Them to Your Life

Cooking the Real Age Way: Turn Back Your Biological Clock
with More than 80 Delicious and Easy Recipes

The RealAge Diet: Make Yourself Younger with What You Eat

RealAge: Are You as Young as You Can Be?

Also by Mehmet C. Oz, M.D.

Healing from the Heart: A Leading Surgeon Combines
Eastern and Western Traditions to Create the Medicine of the Future

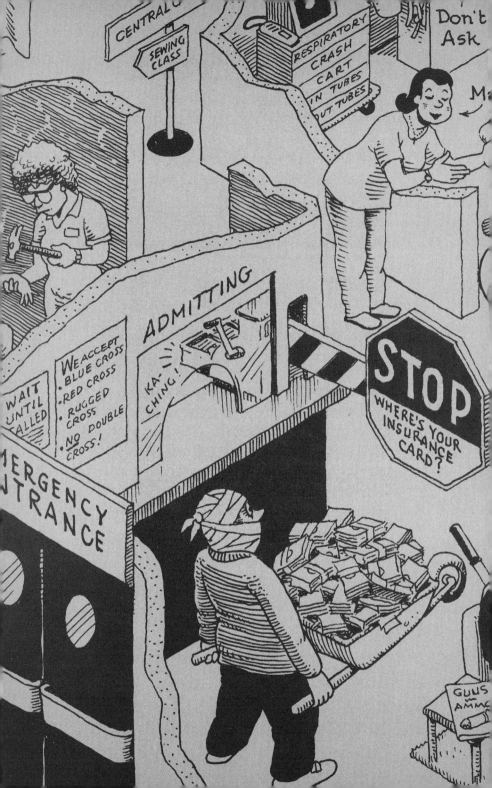

YOU

The Smart Patient

AN INSIDER'S HANDBOOK FOR GETTING THE BEST TREATMENT

• CAUTION • CAUTION • CAUTION •

Michael F. Roizen, M.D.,

and Mehmet C. Oz, M.D.,

with

The Joint Commission
and Joint Commission Resources

and Ron Geraci and Lisa Oz

Illustrations by Gary Hallgren

Free Press
NEW YORK LONDON TORONTO SYDNEY

In certain instances, this book lists Web sites and products by their brand names (such as Web sites you can go to for help and updated information, and medications), because the authors believe that is how this information will be most helpful to you. The authors have also included names of companies and products upon occasion, if they thought that mentioning the name provided relevant information for you. To their knowledge, the authors have no connection to any of the companies, Web sites, or brand-name products listed in the book, with the exception of RealAge, Inc., the company that Mike Roizen helped found for the express purpose of developing the RealAge computer program (www.RealAge.com). Furthermore, the inclusion in this book of any specific commercial products or services provided by any specific individual or company in no way constitutes an endorsement by the authors, the publisher, or the Joint Commission and its affiliates.

Please bear in mind that this book is intended to provide helpful and informative material. The authors are not engaged in rendering medical, health, legal, or any kind of personal professional services in this book, and it should not be considered a substitute for advice from a medical professional or legal counsel. The author and publisher expressly disclaim responsibility for any adverse effects arising from the use or application of the information contained in this book.

FREE PRESS
A Division of Simon & Schuster, Inc.
1230 Avenue of the Americas
New York, NY 10020

Copyright © 2006 by Michael F. Roizen, M.D., and Oz Works LLC, f/s/o
Mehmet C. Oz, M.D., and Joint Commission Resources

All rights reserved,
including the right of reproduction
in whole or in part in any form.

First Free Press trade paperback edition 2006

FREE PRESS and colophon are trademarks
of Simon & Schuster, Inc.

For information regarding special discounts for bulk purchases,
please contact Simon & Schuster Special Sales at 1-800-456-6798
or business@simonandschuster.com

Designed by Ruth Lee Mui

Manufactured in the United States of America

10 9 8 7 6 5 4 3

Library of Congress Cataloging-in-Publication Data is available.

ISBN-13: 978-0-7432-9301-3
ISBN-10:   0-7432-9301-0

To patients and the caregivers who love them

Authors' note

To make this book more enjoyable and useful for you, we have written and illustrated it with a lighthearted and at times even irreverent tone. We hope our colleagues have a sense of humor and understand why we did so.

Make no mistake: we are honored to work in a field that has helped so many people in so many ways. Our colleagues are intensely passionate and compassionate professionals who work hard, and who, like us, are proud of the marvels modern medicine has achieved. But we all also know that medicine is a complex discipline that can be inefficient. We've taken many liberties in depicting exaggerated examples of shortcomings in the health care system, and in creating caricatures of members of the health care community. We ask forgiveness for the poetic license we've employed to bring alive important points in a memorable way.

If anybody should take great offense at the tongue-in-cheek exaggeration in these pages, it's us. Some of the health care system's most vivid failings are blessedly apparent in our daily efforts to treat, heal, serve, and get home in time for a reheated dinner. Mike Roizen is an internist and anesthesiologist; the latter are renowned for practicing their specialty by sitting on a stool and passing gas to patients. Mehmet Oz, like many surgeons, is often in error, but never in doubt. And the Joint Commission on Accreditation of Healthcare Organizations (JCAHO), that feared oversight body, is as cuddly and good humored as any Senate judiciary subcommittee.

Of course, as any reader of the book will see, we have strong opinions on a multitude of subjects, many of which the Joint Commission has not studied and about which it has no official positions. For example, the Joint Commission is not an expert on alternative medicine, insurance, the selection by patients of doctors and hospitals for specific procedures, medication purchasing, and so on.

We only hope the book our motley crew has lovingly produced brings transparency to our sometimes Byzantine health care system. We hope it helps you, and all who follow you, get the best treatment. If it does, the nasty mail and flattened tires will have been worth it. Thanks.

—The Authors

Contents

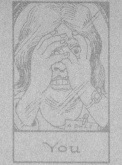

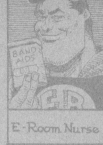

Waiting-room Security

Other Patients

You

E-Room Nurse

Chief Inspector Clouseau

Columbo

Sis

World-renowned

P.I. Kinsey Millhone

Dick Tracy

Neighborhood Pharmacist

Buddy

Resident Doctor

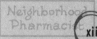

YOU

The Smart Patient

Introduction

Why You Need to Be a Smart Patient

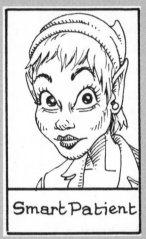

Smart Patient

Midnight. You come home. The door's been forced open. You click on the light, and your worst fear is confirmed. Everything's gone. Your furniture. Your kitchen china. Your autographed Stones album. Your pet hamster Alfredo. In shock and panic, you dash around your violated house with only one thought: how could this have happened? Who knew you were gone? Did you see anyone suspicious? How could the neighbors who notice when you don't cut your grass *not* have noticed the moving van parked in your driveway? And, by God, why did these scoundrels have to leave the ugliest rug in the house?

You call the police. When the detectives finally arrive (cue *Dragnet* theme music), they start firing questions. Where were you? How long were you gone? What's missing? What's not missing? What strange occurrences happened in the last days or weeks? They want the facts, please, just the facts.

After you give them every detail you can, these Columbos start gathering evidence. Fortunately, that tidy contribution you make to the local benevolence association every year is finally paying dividends, and they give you their best no-stone-unturned treatment. They dust for fingerprints. They gingerly tweeze a single strand of strange hair from the brush in the bathroom (those fiends!). They photograph the muddy footprints on the aforementioned rug. The detectives know their mission: they gather the details, find the clues, put 'em all together, and solve the crime. Of course, the detectives combing your house are only a part of the process. If you're ever going to see your penned-up copy of *Let It Bleed* again (let alone your poor asthmatic Alfredo), an entire team of crime solvers must work together to figure who's behind this diabolical act, and how—if there's any chance at all—you might recover what you lost. And though no one may be mentioning it now, there's an even bigger priority than returning you to as good as new; it's most critical to prevent this from ever happening again.

You might be asking, What in the heck does all this have

to do with this book? We hope you are, because having a big propensity to ask questions is the first sign that you're on your way to becoming a Smart Patient.

The finely tuned skills that seasoned police officers use to solve a crime—or, more important, to *prevent* one—are exactly the same skills that the best doctors and patients use to diagnose and treat health problems, and to prevent their recurrence. They gather clues, ask questions, read people, and do efficient legwork, with the help of a partner and other colleagues.

In treating patients every day, we play the part of quasi detectives—though the hospital still hasn't issued us our trench coats and service sidearms, we're miffed to say. Every day, with every patient, we read crime scenes, sift for tiny clues, pursue villains, and search for ways to ensure future security and safety—with the help of our patients. In each investigation, our patient really plays a triple role: he or she is our partner and our chief, and also the very citizen we're protecting and serving.

We recognized this early in our doctoring careers. It gave us more respect for patients than we ever anticipated having when we were in medical school. Of course, not all patients accepted all three duties.

When we began practicing medicine back in the . . . well, some years ago, many patients were still living in the Marcus Welby era. You know, the era when physicians were seen as the supreme authorities. These patients believed everything we said, or pretended to, anyway. They were most comfortable in the day when physicians laid out rigid treatment plans, and patients "followed doctors' orders" or else. We never really needed to go into that "or else" part because patients' imaginations were far more vivid than anything we could cook up.

Other visitors to our humble offices were of a different breed, however. They not only recognized their duties as patients (a.k.a. witnesses), partners, and precinct bosses, they relished taking on these missions. They thrived while challenging us to practice the type of medicine we had always dreamed of practicing, ever since we first listened to our family pooch's heart with a toy stethoscope. It was the kind of medicine in which patients realized the awesome power they had in controlling their own quality of care, and they weren't afraid to use that power to make us better doctors.

These patients knew that our mutual supreme goal—keeping them healthy, strong and in command of their lives—required two sharp brains at a minimum. The best of these patients emerged like golden beacons. We called them by a variety of complimentary names, but most often we referred to them by a highly scientific medical term that suited them best and still does: Smart Patients.

We wrote this handbook in honor of our Smart Patients. We wrote it because we want to see them continue to propagate at an alarming rate. Because we're not fertility specialists or crooners, this book was the best way we could further that cause.

We wrote this book to make *you* a Smart Patient.

Now, that's not to say that you're not already a pretty Smart Patient. In fact, we'll bet you are. (Hey, you could've bought a *Chicken Soup* paperback instead of our book, so that says something right there!) Indeed, you may be the smartest patient we'll ever have the good fortune to see. But the real question is, are you a Smart Patient?

Let's define this term a bit more fully before you answer.

While Smart Patients have existed since Socrates made house calls, we started to see them come into our offices on a regular basis only about ten years ago. That's when some patients began talking about this contraption they found called the Internet. They were using it to teach themselves about medical issues—sometimes accurately, sometimes not. But their numbers increased.

Soon they were hopping on the World Wide Web and learning more about, oh, say, impetigo, in an hour than we remembered after eight years of medical school and residency. Patients began asking about tests and alternative medications that, just a few years ago, were as unknown to them as the art of pygmy pottery was to us. Lines of questioning that had once begun and ended with "What should I do?" now started off with "Do you think I should..." And these questions sometimes included a treatment option that was as intelligent as it was insightful. Occasionally it was even a treatment option that we—physicians, with framed degrees and everything—had not considered.

When that happened, everything changed. Forever.

Marcus Welby had officially retired to his cabin in the woods, not to be seen again. This was the new world order in medicine—one in which empowered patients called the shots and regularly questioned us.

Some doctors hated it.

We loved it.

And we continue to love it more every year, as our roster of Smart Patients happily grows. Smart Patients are ahead of the curve. They come in with specific checklists of tasks for us to do. They know to bring every pill or tablet or chalky powder they take with them when they visit for an appointment. They talk and ask questions and never complain to their spouse that they had wasted their time after sitting like a statue during the appointment—a pet peeve of ours, in case that was too thinly veiled. Smart Patients don't confuse their upcoming cystoscopy with tidbits they've heard about a relative's colonoscopy, which tells us that they actually do know whether they're coming or going.

To be a Smart Patient, you can't be passive; you need to be a first-rate Sherlock Holmes on your problem-solving medical team. Like Holmes, Smart Patients ask intelligent questions and have the instincts (and the guts) to politely challenge things that they don't understand. These qualities may seem elementary, but they're rare—and they are what set Smart Patients apart.

Smart Patients are also practical about their limits. They know they don't need to know all the technical medical details about their health problems, but they need to put at least as much effort into finding out the basics as they did in obtaining the driving directions to our office. They know that we don't always know the answers, but we can join forces with them to find out. Your entire health team—which includes doctors, nurses, specialists, pharmacists, family members, and *you*—works together as savvy detectives charged with interpreting even the tiniest clues to come up with a diagnosis and a treatment plan. And while there's much teamwork in this process, ultimately you are the person most responsible for the success of your health care team. How you explain the facts, how you ask questions, how you educate yourself, and how you lead your health care team will make you a Smart Patient.

While we'd love to take full credit for creating this book, we had some big help.

First and foremost, our Smart Patients taught us much of the info that's contained in these pages. While it's easy to think that a doctor educates his patients (the word doctor comes from a Latin word meaning "teacher"), it's really the other way around with Smart Patients. We stand in awe of them, and we've learned amazing things by working with them—mainly because they make us be the absolute best doctors we can be.

We've also partnered with a group called the Joint Commission on Accreditation of Healthcare Organizations to produce this book. We know, that name is a mouthful. This is probably more than you want to know, but the "Joint," as it's affectionately called by the folks who work there, or Joint Commission by others, is a do-gooder group that makes sure you are safe and getting the best health care possible while on your back undergoing surgery and even while hooked up to machines in intensive care. Chances are extremely good you haven't heard of the Joint Commission. In fact, if you have heard of it, and you don't work in the health care field, we'd be surprised.

But doctors, nurses, hospitals, and everyone else in health care know about the Joint Commission because it delivers what amounts to a report card to care providers who want to give you the best and safest health care. If they live up to these standards, they get accredited—which basically means they meet extremely high standards and safety goals. If a hospital or outpatient clinic or nursing home doesn't work hard to keep you safe and healthy, it won't cut it with the Joint Commission. Sometimes, these facilities are dinged for bad behavior and told to clean up their act. And that's good news for you. Hospitals that don't exercise the utmost care can be treacherous places.

That said, however, even the best facilities make their share of errors. In fact, research shows that you have a 1 in 25 chance of developing a serious unexpected complication (such as a possibly fatal infection) when you check into the hospital. Those odds don't sound terrifying? Consider that you'll probably check into the hospital for various treatments at least five or six times in your life. That means your odds of being affected by that potentially deadly, unforeseen complication might be as high as 2 in 5. An even more frightening statistic? Seventy-five percent of these complications are *completely preventable.*

Restated, the odds that you'll need to use the tips in this book to save your life or for critical well-being are shockingly good. If you're a gambler, it would be the smart bet. In surveys, nearly half of all Americans say they have been touched by medical errors.

Now, all the above odds and statistics may not be familiar, but you've probably heard some of these often-stated numbers before. All tallied, medical mistakes in U.S. hospitals alone cause an estimated 44,000 to 98,000 fatalities a year. (You can see what a slippery problem this is; we can't even nail down a true number.) But even if you take the lower figure, that's 120 deaths a day; this is far more than twice the number claimed by drunk driving. Even breast cancer claims fewer lives, while provoking far more attention. Nonfatal but damaging mistakes likely number in the hundreds of thousands per year. Checking into the hospital for "routine surgery" (a pairing as logical as "nonalcoholic gin") is not as dangerous as, say, running onto the racetrack during the Indy 500 and trying to traverse the traffic with a pogo stick. But it's closer to it than we'd like.

In addition to the doctors, nurses, and thousands of other health care pros toiling on the front lines every day, the Joint Commission is one of the behind-the-scenes players working to improve patient safety. The Joint Commission used to tell hospitals and other providers when its agents were going to visit and "survey" them (read: check up on them to see if they're doing the job right). As you can imagine, the hospital or outpatient clinic never looked better than the night before the Joint Commission showed up. But in an effort to be more relevant and effective, the Joint Commission's surveyors now show up unannounced. These inspections catch conditions that are a little closer to day-to-day reality. The Joint Commission has rules about medications, surgery, patient safety, cleanliness to prevent infections, and so on—stuff you probably don't even want to think about. It is often an unpopular watchdog (that's good for you) that's not afraid to show its teeth when it needs to, and what shiny, sharp teeth the Joint has.

Finally, we know a picture is worth a million shrewd questions, so we've packed our book chock-full of visual clues for your forensic benefit (and pleasure). Specifically, we've included mug shots of the suspects and characters you'll meet in every situation we describe in the upcoming chapters, as well as painstakingly detailed (if not always literal) renditions of scenes you may encounter. Use the smarts acquired by reading *You: The Smart Patient*, and your own experiences with the health care system won't be nearly as harrowing as those depicted in the pages ahead. We promise.

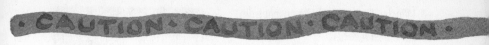
THE SMART PATIENT QUIZ

Surprise!

Pop quiz.

To help you gauge how much you really know about taking control of your health care, sharpen a No. 2 pencil (or a No. 3, if you're the kind who never follows rules) and take a shot at answering the following questions. It won't take you but a few minutes. The answers start on page 23.

1. What's the most important thing to bring with you to the doctor's office?

    a. A properly completed living will, to be kept on file

    b. Your husband or wife

    c. A crisp $50 bill in an envelope

    d. An accurate and complete health profile

    e. A photo of yourself at age twelve

2. When giving your doctor your family history, which tidbit below would be most critical to mention?

    a. My uncle had asbestosis and needed oxygen when he was seventy.

    b. My mother is so healthy she beats up the neighbors.

    c. My husband smokes.

    d. My father is becoming forgetful now that he's 88.

    e. My brother is a 440-pound diabetic.

3. Which will most likely be absent from your medical records?

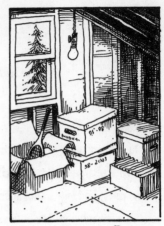

Home Records Room

   a. The scribbled note regarding a tetanus shot you received in 1972
   b. The pathology report from that "thing" you had removed twelve years ago
   c. X-rays from your father's quadruple bypass surgery before he turned sixty-five
   d. Notes on your "bad attitude and know-it-all disposition" from a doctor whom you don't even remember seeing
   e. Photocopies of random things that make no sense whatsoever

4. Your doctor says you need to undergo a medical diagnostic test. Which question should you definitely ask first?

   a. How accurate is this test?
   b. What exactly does this test measure?
   c. Why do you think I need this test, and what'll happen if I don't take it?
   d. Who is going to pay for this?
   e. Will the probe that's used in this test be brand-new?

5. Board certification means:

   a. A doctor has served in a managerial position at a large hospital.
   b. A doctor is extremely physically fit.
   c. A doctor is skilled in treating lumber.
   d. A doctor had to study under a specialist for a period of eight years.
   e. A doctor passed several exams showing specialized skill.

6. A hospitalist is

    a. A patient who checks into the hospital for every little ailment

    b. A doctor who works only in hospitals and has no private practice

    c. A medical professional who rates the quality of hospitals

    d. A shorthand term for a list of hospitals

    e. A nurse who splits his or her time among two different hospitals

7. When is the best time to schedule a doctor appointment?

    a. In the early afternoon on Friday

    b. Weekends, since all the other patients are enjoying themselves

    c. In the late morning, after your doctor has had his coffee

    d. The first appointment of the day, whenever that is

    e. Any time on Wednesday, which is traditionally a slow day for doctors

8. Prior to entering the operating room, you should

    a. Shave and clean the surgical site to help prevent an infection

    b. Make sure you're wearing clean underwear

    c. Pray, even if you're an atheist

    d. Make sure you strip off your nail polish

    e. Ask the surgeon to make sure that the surgical instruments have been properly sterilized

9. Which of the following is the least important quality in finding a great hospital?

    a. It should be close enough to your home area so friends can visit, which is important for your morale.

    b. It should be able to prove that it performs high numbers of the procedure you need done.

   c. The hospital should have high marks for quality in state databases.

   d. The hospital's managerial staff should all be practicing, board-certified doctors.

   e. The emergency room should have a policy of not charging anyone who comes in on his birthday.

10. Which of the following medical professionals should you ask for recommendations for a surgeon?

   a. An anesthesiologist

   b. Your doctor's billing manager

   c. A homeopathic practitioner

   d. Your local paramedics

   e. None of the above

11. If you're going to undergo heart bypass surgery, you should go to a hospital that performs at least this many such procedures per year:

   a. 5 (but they're all perfect)

   b. 50

   c. 500

   d. 5,000

   e. It doesn't matter, as long as the surgeon is extremely skilled in the operation.

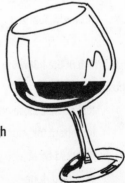

12. Which of the following should you always ask for before surgery?

   a. Carbohydrates, so your blood sugar remains high

   b. A blanket

   c. A sip of brandy

d. The credentials of your surgeon's assisting staff

e. A mud facial

13. The most accessible and least expensive health care resource you have is:

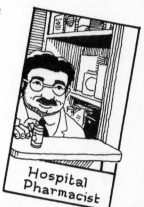

a. Google.com

b. The nurse hotlines provided by some health insurers

c. Your pharmacist

d. The self-help section at the local bookstore

e. Your neighbor's fortune-teller

Hospital Pharmacist

14. Which question should you ask your doctor when he or she is writing you a new prescription?

a. Good grief, what are these scribbles supposed to say?

b. Any chance you could write me a script for a generic version, so I can save some money?

c. Is this replacing any of the other pills I'm taking?

d. Can I take this pill with my morning grapefruit juice?

e. All of the above

15. Which of the following should you think twice about before asking your pharmacist?

a. Do you have a computer system that'll prevent a serious mix-up in my meds?

b. I can get these pills down the block for twenty bucks less. Can you beat that price?

c. What kind of deal do I get if I buy in bulk?

d. Only the last two statements

e. None of the above

16. Your prescription note reads *prn.* What does that mean?

a. This medication is for a prenatal condition.

b. You should take the drug during the day, prior to nighttime.

c. You should take this medication only before watching an adult film.

d. You should take the pills on alternate days.

e. You should take the pills as needed.

17. The best ER

a. Is a dead ER

b. Offers round-the-clock MRI testing

c. Has less than a two-hour average wait

d. Resembles Woodstock only on Saturday nights

e. Is disinfected by professional cleaners every six hours

18. A level-three emergency room is:

a. An ER staffed by doctors, nurses, and pharmacists

b. An ER on the third floor of the hospital

c. An ER with the fewest capabilities

d. An ER with the greatest capabilities

e. An ER that treats at least three gunshot victims a week

19. In choosing a hospital, which criterion below is the only one you shouldn't insist on?

a. The hospital has a strong connection with your primary-care doctor.

b. The hospital has a relationship with your insurance company.

c. The hospital is accredited by the Joint Commission.

16

d. The hospital has an appropriate ratio of resident doctors to experienced doctors.

e. The nurses aren't hopelessly overworked.

20. Where should you sit in the ER waiting room?

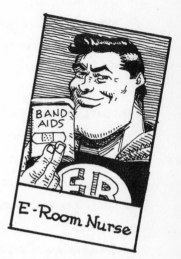

E-Room Nurse

a. On the seat closest to the ER nurse so he notices you

b. Anywhere but near the vending machines

c. On a plastic chair rather than a cloth chair

d. On a pillow, because you're going to be there for at least twenty-two hours, most likely

e. In earshot of the double doors leading to the treatment areas, so your moaning and wailing will not go unheeded

21. The number of preventable hospital deaths per year is about equal to:

a. The deaths of all American soldiers in Vietnam

b. The deaths from motor vehicle accidents in America annually

c. The deaths from HIV (human immunodeficiency virus) in a year

d. The deaths from diabetes in a year

e. All of the above combined

22. Which words do you ideally want to characterize your hospital stay?

a. Slow and methodical

b. Informative and poignant

c. Boring and short

d. Life changing and eye opening

e. Cheaper than anticipated

23. The biggest enemy you have in your hospital room is:
    a. The guy who comes to collect cash for the television service
    b. The least experienced doctor who may conceivably treat you during the course of your stay
    c. Your phone-addicted roommate
    d. The germs in the room
    e. The billing clerk

24. The best protection against hospital infections is:
    a. Making visitors wear masks
    b. Taking 10,000 milligrams (mg) of vitamin C each day
    c. Paying extra for a private room
    d. Being obsessive about asking every person who treats you to wash his or her hands
    e. Going to a hospital in a high-altitude area, such as Denver

25. The most germ-ridden object in your hospital room is:
    a. The flush handle on the throne
    b. The food tray
    c. The doorknob
    d. The TV remote control
    e. You

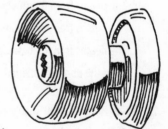

26. During which of the following periods should you avoid checking into the hospital, if you can?
    a. The holiday season
    b. Midsummer

    c. Full moons

    d. Oscar night

    e. The days right after a good, hard rain

27. What two-word utterance used to cause greater tension between doctors and patients than the words "I'll sue"?

    a. "No insurance"

    b. "Big fingers"

    c. They rhyme with *duck* and *moo*

    d. "Second opinion"

    e. "Joint Commission"

28. How often does getting a second opinion change treatment substantially?

    a. In about one-third of all cases

    b. In about 20 percent of all cases

    c. In about 60 percent of all cases

    d. Very rarely, surprisingly

    e. What's a second opinion?

29. If a doctor gives you a troubling diagnosis, you should ask all but which one of the following questions?

    a. Who, other than you, is the best physician at treating this?

    b. Are there any clinical trials sponsored by National Institutes of Health underway for this condition or disease?

    c. What are the odds that this diagnosis is incorrect?

    d. Will you still treat me if I get a second opinion?

    e. Will this condition affect my golf game in any way, shape, or form?

30. How many rights do you have when you check into a hospital?

    a. Roughly as many as you would have in a jail cell

    b. None, if your doctor writes *"no rights"* on your paperwork

    c. More than you would probably believe

    d. Six

    e. Depends on how wealthy you are, frankly

31. Which of the following are you guaranteed when you check into a hospital?

    a. Your fanny will stick out of the hospital gown.

    b. You'll be given full disclosure of all costs.

    c. Your hospital bill will be explained to you so you can understand it.

    d. You'll wonder why the $3,000-a-day fee doesn't get you better food.

    e. You'll receive speedy and dignified care, at least in theory.

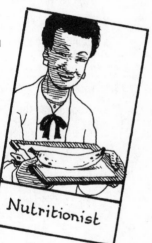

Nutritionist

32. What is the Health Insurance Portability and Accountability Act (HIPAA)?

    a. It's a law that ensures that you can take your health-insurance policy to any state in the U.S.

    b. It's a piece of legislation that protects the confidentiality of your medical records.

    c. It forces all insurers to issue you, upon request, cards with magnetic strips that store all of your health-insurance information, so it's always handy.

    d. It's a law that guarantees that people who commit insurance fraud and flee to foreign countries will be pursued, extradited, and prosecuted.

e. It's a law that makes physicians everywhere rejoice and say, "It's about time!"

33. If you consent to become someone's "health care proxy," what have you just agreed to do?
   a. To visit her doctors on her behalf if she's traveling or otherwise indisposed
   b. To take her medications, too, to see if any side effects show up in both of you
   c. To pay her medical bills if she cannot
   d. To ensure that the stipulations listed in her living will are followed
   e. To give her bone marrow or part of your liver if the need arises

34. What is the main benefit of participating in a medical study?
   a. They generally pay well.
   b. The food is free.
   c. You have a much reduced risk of side effects or complications, since you're being watched so closely.
   d. You'll get meticulous care, albeit possibly with unproven therapies.
   e. The monogrammed bowling shirt.

35. Fifty billion dollars is:
   a. The cost of all medical care in Canada
   b. The amount Hollywood starlets spend annually on plastic surgery
   c. The yearly out-of-pocket health care expenditures for all Americans
   d. What Americans spend on alternative medicine treatments per year
   e. The winnings of the best malpractice law firm in the year 2005

36. What is the difference between the ginseng and the prescription medication sitting side by side on your nightstand?

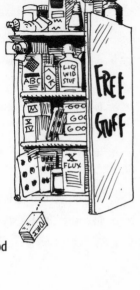

 a. Actually, very little

 b. Your doctor probably had a free sample of the ginseng

 c. About the difference between a mutt and a pedigreed show dog

 d. Your insurance company would rather you try the first before the second

 e. All of the above

37. Who is the best person to find out about how good an insurance company is at handling your claims?

 a. Your doctor's or hospital's billing guru

 b. Your doctor

 c. The human resources representative at your company

 d. The Joint Commission

 e. The Better Business Bureau in your state

38. What is the biggest advantage most HMO insurance plans have over current indemnity health-insurance plans?

 a. Docs and hospitals relish dealing with the HMO billing computers.

 b. The indemnity plan will cost you less over the course of the year.

 c. The HMO is generally more focused on paying for needed treatment, while indemnity plans are more focused on preventing illnesses.

 d. The HMO is cheaper, because it bargains with doctors and hospitals to reduce costs by as much as 80 percent.

 e. The HMO provides a complaint hotline.

39. Which statement will likely get the biggest reaction from your insurance company when you're trying to resolve a dispute?

    a. "I'm going to phone your CEO!"

    b. "I'm going to report you to the Better Business Bureau!"

    c. "You can expect a personal call from my physician!"

    d. "I'm going to contact the state insurance commissioner!"

    e. "My lawyer has a 90 percent victory record in insurance cases!"

40. If you appeal a claim denial from your health-insurance company, what are the odds that you'll get the insurer to reverse its decision?

    a. About 1 in 4; roughly 25 percent of appeals are successful

    b. 1 in 12; with a little luck, it could happen

    c. 1 in 2; your odds are excellent

    d. About 1 in 7 if you threaten to involve the state insurance commissioner

    e. About 1 in 6 if you *are* the state insurance commissioner

Finished? Great. Here are the answers.

1. What's the most important thing to bring with you to the doctor's office?

    a. A properly completed living will, to be kept on file

    b. Your husband or wife

    c. A crisp $50 bill in an envelope

    d. An accurate and complete health profile

    e. A photo of yourself at age twelve

That's right, *d.* Bringing your complete health profile is the most valuable thing you can have in tow, even above your precious insurance card. In chapter one, we'll show you the exact information you need to have handy.

2. When giving your doctor your family history, which tidbit below would be most critical to mention?

    a. My uncle had asbestosis and needed oxygen when he was seventy.

    b. My mother is so healthy she beats up the neighbors.

    c. My husband smokes.

    d. My father is becoming forgetful now that he's 88.

    e. My brother is a 440-pound diabetic.

Even though your spouse isn't a blood relative, his daily bad habits can be a bigger risk to your health much more than expected, common, or lifestyle-caused risk factors in your blood kin—which most of the above examples illustrate.

3. Which will most likely be absent from your medical records?

    a. The scribbled note regarding a tetanus shot you received in 1972

    b. The pathology report from that "thing" you had removed twelve years ago

    c. X-rays from your father's quadruple bypass surgery before he turned sixty-five

    d. Notes on your "bad attitude and know-it-all disposition" from a doctor whom you don't even remember seeing

    e. Photocopies of random things that make no sense whatsoever

You'll likely find everything in that mishmash of information pertaining to you, but nothing about your family. That is unfortunate, since the specific information regarding your relative's significant problems can mean a ton to your own health.

4. Your doctor says you need to undergo a medical diagnostic test. Which question should you definitely ask first?

    a. How accurate is this test?

    b. What exactly does this test measure?

24

    c. Who is going to pay for this?

    d. Why do you think I need this test, and what'll happen if I don't take it?

    e. Will the probe that's used in this test be brand new?

That's question number one.

5. Board certification means:

    a. A doctor has served in a managerial position at a large hospital.

    b. A doctor is extremely physically fit.

    c. A doctor is skilled in working with lumber.

    d. A doctor had to study under a specialist for a period of eight years.

    e. A doctor passed several exams in a specialized area.

And he has to receive continuing education in that area to keep his board certification as well, so that's a credential to look for—whether it's board certification in pediatrics, dermatology, or the dozens of other areas.

6. A hospitalist is

    a. A patient who checks into the hospital for every little ailment

    b. A doctor who works only in hospitals and has no private practice

    c. A medical professional who rates the quality of hospitals

    d. A shorthand term for a list of hospitals

    e. A nurse who splits his or her time among two different hospitals

These doctors can be very valuable when you're facing a hospital stay, given their specialized training.

7. When is the best time to schedule a doctor appointment?

   a. In the early afternoon on Friday

   b. Weekends, since all the other patients are enjoying themselves

   c. In the late morning, after your doctor has had his coffee

   d. The first appointment of the day, whenever that is

   e. Any time on Wednesday, which is traditionally a slow day for doctors

Grab that first appointment, before things get monstrously backed up!

8. Prior to entering the operating room, you should

   a. Shave and clean the surgical site to help prevent an infection

   b. Make sure you're wearing clean underwear

   c. Pray, even if you're an atheist

   d. Make sure you strip off your nail polish

   e. Ask the surgeon to make sure that the surgical instruments have been properly sterilized

It's *d*, no kidding. You need to enter the OR the way you entered the world: without any makeup, polish, or piercings that can get in the way, harbor germs, or end up sewn inside you. Shaving your surgical site? That's a common mistake, one that causes many hospital infections. Skip to chapter 3 if you have surgery coming up.

9. Which of the following is the least important quality in finding a great hospital?

   a. It should be close enough to your home area so friends can visit, which is important to your morale.

   b. It should be able to prove that it performs high numbers of the procedure you need done.

c. The hospital should have high marks for quality in state databases.

d. The hospital's managerial staff should all be practicing, board-certified doctors.

e. The emergency room should have a policy of not charging anyone who comes in on his birthday.

People drive farther to get cheap groceries than they do to get the best medical care! If the best hospital is nine hours away, go there if you can. Visitors are great, but highly optional.

10. Which of the following medical professionals should you ask for recommendations for a surgeon?

a. An anesthesiologist

b. Your doctor's billing manager

c. A homeopathic practitioner

d. Your local paramedics

e. None of the above

You can certainly ask 'em all, and they may have a good referral for you. But always hit your hospital's anesthesiologist. The knockout guys see all of the surgeons in action.

11. If you're going to undergo heart bypass surgery, you should go to a hospital that performs at least this many such procedures per year:

a. 5 (but they're all perfect)

b. 50

c. 500

d. 5,000

e. It doesn't matter, as long as the surgeon is extremely skilled in the operation.

Five hundred is the magic number for heart operations, but the minimum number of times a hospital should perform a certain procedure or surgery per year to show competency varies with each kind of procedure. See chapter 3 to learn more of this must-know info.

12. Which of the following should you always ask for before surgery?

    a. Carbohydrates, so your blood sugar remains high

    b. A blanket

    c. A sip of brandy

    d. The credentials of your surgeon's assisting staff

    e. A mud facial

Being cold during surgery can lower your resistance to infection.

13. The most accessible and least expensive health care resource you have is:

    a. Google.com

    b. The nurse hotlines provided by some health insurers

    c. Your pharmacist

    d. The self-help section at the local bookstore

    e. Your neighbor's fortune-teller

You'll see why in chapter 4.

14. Which question should you ask your doctor when he or she is writing you a new prescription?

    a. Good grief, what are these scribbles supposed to say?

    b. Any chance you could write me a script for a generic version, so I can save some money?

    c. Is this replacing any of the other pills I'm taking?

    d. Can I take this pill with my morning grapefruit juice?

    e. All of the above

They're all legit questions. More than legit, they could save your life, or your sacred fortune over time.

15. Which of the following should you think twice about before asking your pharmacist?

    a. Do you have a computer system that'll prevent a serious mix-up in my meds?

    b. I can get these pills down the block for twenty bucks less. Can you beat that price?

    c. What kind of deal do I get if I buy in bulk?

    d. Only the last two statements

    e. None of the above

You need to know if the pharmacist has a cutting-edge safety system, since it can be critical to your protection. And what about asking for discounts? Sure. Why not? A pharmacy is a business, pure and simple.

16. Your prescription note reads *prn.* What does that mean?

    a. This medication is for a prenatal condition.

    b. You should take the drug during the day, prior to nighttime.

    c. You should take this medication only before watching an adult film.

    d. You should take the pills on alternate days.

    e. You should take the pills as needed.

That's right, it means take it only as needed. The abbreviation *prn* is short for *pro re nata,* which is Latin for "the thing that has arisen," which came to mean "as needed" or "as required" in the doctoring lexicon. You'd think that by now we could forgo the Latin and abbreviate it to *a.n.* or *a.r.,* but perhaps that would make things too *persimplicis.* Learn the prescription jargon (on page 141 in chapter 4) so you'll know if your pharmacist read the prescription correctly. That bottle label is only as reliable as the person who typed it—and people make mistakes.

17. The best ER:
   a. Is a dead ER
   b. Offers round-the-clock MRI testing
   c. Has less than a two-hour average wait
   d. Resembles Woodstock only on Saturday nights
   e. Is disinfected by professional cleaners every six hours

The capability to do round-the-clock diagnostic testing is an important mark of a great emergency room; you don't want to wait half a day for the results of tests like these when your life could depend on quick answers.

18. A level-three emergency room is:
   a. An ER where all of the doctors are also board-certified in pediatrics
   b. An ER on the third floor of the hospital
   c. An ER with the fewest capabilities
   d. An ER with the greatest capabilities
   e. An ER that treats at least three gunshot victims a week

Did you know that emergency rooms are rated as one-, two-, and three-level facilities? You do now. And that knowledge could make all the difference one eventful day.

19. In choosing a hospital, which criterion below is the only one you shouldn't insist on?

    a. The hospital has a strong connection with your primary care doctor.

    b. The hospital has a relationship with your insurance company.

    c. The hospital is accredited by the Joint Commission.

    d. The hospital has an appropriate ratio of resident doctors to experienced doctors.

    e. The nurses aren't hopelessly overworked.

Hey, new doctors can be handy, but their ratio to experienced doctors isn't a primary concern. The other factors are musts, however.

20. Where should you sit in the ER waiting room?

    a. On the seat closest to the ER nurse so he notices you

    b. Anywhere but near the vending machines

    c. On a plastic chair rather than a cloth chair

    d. On a pillow, because you're going to be there for at least twenty-two hours, most likely

    e. In earshot of the double doors leading to the treatment areas, so your moaning and wailing will not go unheeded

Plastic is easier to clean, and in an ER, that matters.

21. The number of preventable hospital deaths per year is about equal to:

    a. The deaths of all American soldiers in Vietnam

    b. The deaths from motor vehicle accidents in America annually

    c. The deaths from HIV in a year

    d. The deaths from diabetes in a year

    e. All of the above combined

It's estimated that as many as 98,000 patients die every year due to errors in hospitals.

22. Which words do you ideally want to characterize your hospital stay?
    a. Slow and methodical
    b. Informative and poignant
    c. **Boring and short**
    d. Life changing and eye opening
    e. Cheaper than anticipated

Boring and short means you avoided all of those exciting, life-endangering complications and got out before a germ could infect you. Ho-hum is what you want.

23. The biggest enemy you have in your hospital room is:
    a. The guy who comes to collect cash for the television service
    b. The least experienced doctor who may conceivably treat you during the course of your stay
    c. Your phone-addicted roommate
    d. **The germs in the room**
    e. The billing clerk

Hospital infections from germs such as *B staphylococcus, klebsiella, enterobacter,* and *E. coli* cause as many as 90,000 patients to die every year.

24. The best protection against hospital infections is:
    a. Making visitors wear masks
    b. Taking 10,000 mg of vitamin C each day

   c. Paying extra for a private room

d. Being obsessive about asking every person who treats you to wash his or her hands

   e. Going to a hospital in a high-altitude area, such as Denver

Scrub-a-dub-dub. See chapter 6 for all the dirt on why this is a non-negotiable move.

25. The most germ-ridden object in your hospital room is:

   a. The flush handle on the throne

   b. The food tray

   c. The doorknob

d. The TV remote control

   e. You

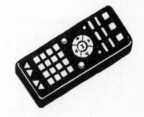

It's the filthiest thing in the room! See chapter 6 for more on this.

26. During which of the following periods should you avoid checking into the hospital, if you can?

   a. The holiday season

b. Midsummer

   c. Full moons

   d. Oscar night

   e. The days right after a good, hard rain

New doctors start their jobs in July, so the hospital is crawling with newbies trying to learn their way around the halls. Give them a few months to break in.

27. What two-word utterance used to cause greater tension between doctors and patients than the words "I'll sue"?

    a. "No insurance"

    b. "Big fingers"

    c. They rhyme with *duck* and *moo*

    d. "Second opinion"

    e. "Joint Commission"

Once, but no more, fortunately.

28. How often does getting a second opinion change treatment substantially?

    a. In about one-third of all cases

    b. In about 20 percent of all cases

    c. In about 60 percent of all cases

    d. Very rarely, surprisingly

    e. What's a second opinion?

This makes it all the more amazing that so few patients get second opinions. Smart Patients never forgo them, because they know facts like this.

29. If a doctor gives you a troubling diagnosis, you should ask all but which one of the following questions?

    a. Who, other than you, is the best physician at treating this?

    b. Are there any clinical trials sponsored by National Institutes of Health underway for this condition or disease?

    c. What are the odds that this diagnosis is incorrect?

    d. Will you still treat me if I get a second opinion?

    e. Will this condition affect my golf game in any way, shape, or form?

This question went out with eight-track tapes. Doctors expect you to get a second opinion for serious health issues; they certainly would if they were sick.

30. How many rights do you have when you check into a hospital?
    a. Roughly as many as you would have in a jail cell
    b. None, if your doctor writes "no rights" on your paperwork
    c. More than you would probably believe
    d. Six
    e. Depends on how wealthy you are, frankly

You have dozens of rights that you probably never even imagined. But it's up to you to use them.

31. Which of the following are you guaranteed when you check into a hospital?
    a. Your fanny will stick out of the hospital gown.
    b. You'll be given full disclosure of all costs.
    c. Your hospital bill will be explained to you so you can understand it.
    d. You'll wonder why the $3,000-a-day fee doesn't get you better food.
    e. You'll receive speedy and dignified care, at least in theory.

First the hospital would have to find someone who could decipher the thing, and that could take days. But this is one of your rights.

32. What is the Health Insurance Portability and Accountability Act (HIPAA)?
    a. It's a law that ensures that you can take your health-insurance policy to any state in the U.S.
    b. It's a piece of legislation that protects the confidentiality of your medical records.

c. It forces all insurers to issue you, upon request, cards with magnetic strips that store all of your health-insurance information, so it's always handy.

d. It's a law that guarantees that people who commit insurance fraud and flee to foreign countries will be pursued, extradited, and prosecuted.

e. It's a law that makes physicians everywhere rejoice and say, "It's about time!"

HIPAA protects your confidentiality but makes it a lot harder for doctors to access and share necessary information about you too.

33. If you consent to become someone's "health care proxy," what have you just agreed to do?
   a. To visit her doctors on her behalf if she's traveling or otherwise indisposed
   b. To take her medications too, to see if any side effects show up in both of you
   c. To pay her medical bills if she cannot.
   d. To ensure that the stipulations listed in her living will are followed
   e. To give her bone marrow or part of your liver if the need arises

Do you have an appointed health care proxy? If not, why not? Chapter 8 will explain why this is more important than you likely believe.

34. What is the main benefit of participating in a medical study?
   a. They generally pay well.
   b. The food is free.
   c. You have a much reduced risk of side effects or complications, since you're being watched so closely.
   d. You'll get meticulous care, albeit possibly with unproven therapies.
   e. The monogrammed bowling shirt.

Sure, it might be unproven, but it could also save your life.

35. Fifty billion dollars is:

    a. The cost of all medical care in Canada

    b. The amount Hollywood starlets spend annually on plastic surgery

    c. What Americans spend on alternative medicine treatments per year

    d. The yearly out-of-pocket health care expenditures for all Americans

    e. The winnings of the best malpractice law firm in the year 2005

The answers are *c* and *d.* No joke. We'll explain the good, bad, and funky of this phenomenon in chapter 9.

36. What is the difference between the ginseng and the prescription medication sitting side by side on your nightstand?

    a. Actually, very little

    b. Your doctor probably had a free sample of the ginseng

    c. About the difference between a mutt and a pedigree show dog

    d. Your insurance company would rather you try the first before the second

    e. All of the above

Herbal supplements aren't tested by the FDA for quality and don't always contain what their labels claim, unlike heavily regulated prescription drugs. Those ginseng tablets may have almost no ginseng in them—unless there's a "UPS-verified" mark on the bottle. See chapter 9 for an explanation of why.

37. Who is the best person to find out about how good an insurance company is at handling your claims?

    a. Your doctor's or hospital's billing guru

    b. Your doctor

    c. The human resources representative at your company

    d. The Joint Commission

    e. The Better Business Bureau in your state

She deals with the vagaries of insurance claims every day, and she knows who pays up right away and who holds back those checks for months.

38. What is the biggest advantage most HMO insurance plans have over current indemnity health-insurance plans?

    a. Doctors and hospitals relish dealing with the HMO billing computers.

    b. The indemnity plan will cost you less over the course of the year.

    c. The HMO is generally more focused on paying for needed treatment, while indemnity plans are more focused on preventing illnesses.

    d. The HMO is cheaper, because it bargains with doctors and hospitals to reduce costs by as much as 80 percent.

    e. The HMO provides a complaint hotline.

By guaranteeing a large amount of exclusive business to specific doctors and hospitals, HMOs can twist arms to get colossal pricing discounts.

39. Which statement will likely get the biggest reaction from your insurance company when you're trying to resolve a dispute?

    a. "I'm going to phone your CEO!"

    b. "I'm going to report you to the Better Business Bureau!"

    c. "You can expect a personal call from my physician!"

    d. "I'm going to contact the state insurance commissioner!"

    e. My lawyer has a 90 percent victory record in insurance cases!"

The insurance commissioner is the big kahuna to the insurers, so dropping that bomb—should it become necessary—can help you prevail in a disagreement. But it's certainly not the ideal opening blow; see chapter 8 for the smartest route to get what you need.

40. If you appeal a claim denial from your health-insurance company, what are the odds that you'll get the insurer to reverse its decision?
  a. About 1 in 4; roughly 25 percent of appeals are successful.
  b. 1 in 12; with a little luck, it could happen.
  c. 1 in 2; your odds are excellent
  d. About 1 in 7 if you threaten to involve the state insurance commissioner.
  e. About 1 in 6 if you *are* the state insurance commissioner.

According to research, you have about a 50 percent chance of winning an appeal. Persistence is going to be key, as we'll reveal.

So, How Did You Do?

If you missed only one to five answers, you're at the head of the class. Congratulations!

If you missed five to ten answers, you have the ready makings of a Smart Patient; read chapters 4, 7, 8, and 10 first to bone up on the information you're most likely lacking, and then hit the rest of the chapters to get the advanced insider info that only elite Smart Patients know.

You missed more than ten? Well, you're one of them: the new and soon-to-be Smart Patients. Take ten chapters of highly potent tips in convenient daily doses and supplement with the appendices as needed. You'll be at the peak of your Smart Patient powers in no time. And that's a powerful way to ensure that you—and your significant others, as well as anyone you'll influence by reading *You: The Smart Patient*—will stay in peak health for all of your years to come.

1
Getting to Know You

Let's Discover the Juicy Secrets
About the Person Who Controls Your Health: You

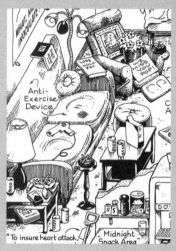

Most people think they communicate with their doctors just fine. Better than fine, in fact. Fantastic. Given that most of the communication consists of nodding or a request for antibiotics, there's little to find fault with. That's the problem, of course. Most patients don't do a great job of communicating with their doctors because patients often give us too little pertinent information to go on (remember, just like the detective, we're looking for the facts). At the same time, they may also give us too many distracting or off-topic details. It reminds us a little bit of what a mechanic must think when we try to explain a noise in our car. We're not sure when it started, we're not sure what makes it worse, we think it's a whining sound but aren't sure . . . We bet this becomes a tedious monologue for those earnest professionals trying to help us.

An almost identical conversation goes on in doctors' offices every day. To be accurate, the parallel exchanges often concern befuddled male patients. There's a reason that women aged thirty to sixty are the prime decision makers about health care in the United States. Most of the guys they love either have no clue about their health needs or wouldn't see a doctor unless they had blood shooting out of both ears.

The goal of this chapter is to make sure you know the details and numbers in your health profile that you really need to know—those stats and specifics that are crucial to you and your doctor. We always see health books and well-intentioned magazine articles that tell you to compile so much stuff, we get winded just reading the list. The average person would have to take a week off from work and probably hire a bounty hunter to get everything recommended. You don't need to do that, but you do need to assemble a thorough health history so that you'll have a body of evidence to use when working with your doctor. A big part of being a Smart Patient is knowing how to compare new evidence (such as new test results) against the old. Like Sherlock Holmes, even though something may seem elementary to everyone else and not worth asking about, you need to press on with your questions and your investigation.

We'll make compiling your health history simple enough to do, but we won't oversimplify the tasks so you lose accuracy. It's a small time investment that could save your life, so get started right away.

You Love Us? Ditto

The first sign of a Smart Patient is that telltale document they produce during their first visit, or even their fiftieth. It's a portent of a beautiful partnership—that is, when it's not a form they need signed for their job, or a note asking one of our office assistants about their dinner plans. If we're lucky, it'll be their health profile. It's the sign of a patient who means business, one who will challenge us to be at our absolute best and who won't waste time and money on redundant and unnecessary efforts (which can lead to errors). To create the perfect health profile, circa early twenty-first century, flip ahead to appendix 2, Sample Forms, and find the forms labeled **Your Health Journal.** Make copies of them, or rip them out if that's handier. The forms are also online at **www.jcrinc.com** and **www.realage.com.**

Fill them out.

Finished? Everything? You're done. That is, if you don't have any questions, and you're sure it's all correct. Just bring those forms to your doctor along with a baggie filled with

Sherlock Holmes & Dr. Watson

every medication, vitamin, herb, or whatever else you take regularly (in their original bottles). Store copies of the forms in a fireproof safe, and update them yearly or whenever a piece of key info changes. Everyone's happy.

What's that? It wasn't that simple? You don't know all the info by heart or have it filed neatly in your credenza? Now, that's woefully human of you. If you're like most of our patients, you've never compiled your important health info before, and you may not have the foggiest notion of where to find much of it—or even if it exists at all. Even with using the forms as guides, your records may be so scattered that you don't know where to start.

Let's take it from the beginning.

Start in Top Form

Fill out all the easy stuff on the forms labeled **Your Health Journal**, such as your birth date, address, your doctor's contact info, your pharmacy, your insurance info, and everything else listed. As you may suspect, this will be your master form, the one you perhaps store on your computer, and give out whenever necessary, including when you visit a new medical professional or step foot in a hospital. (Take at least two copies, and always give one to the admitting nurse who welcomes you to your bed.)

This form won't just make your life easier, it'll prevent a severe case of hand cramps from rewriting half of this info dozens of times in the future. And bypassing twenty occasions that require you to blearily check boxes before you've had your morning coffee (and having another fallible person decipher that scrawl) is a no-brainer way of reducing errors.

Under the section entitled Your Health Now, write down every significant ailment or condition that you have *right now*. This would be the place to list ongoing conditions such as diabetes, hypertension, psoriasis, depression, back pain, and the like. Don't include anything you had years ago but don't have now; that goes in a different place. Be certain to include anything that you're taking medication for, even if the specific symptoms are gone; for example, if you're controlling your high blood pressure with medication, list high blood pressure. Next to each condition, list when you were diagnosed, what medication you're taking for it, if any, and any other relevant info. If you're not sure if it's relevant, jot it down. That's why your doctor's office assistant has Wite-Out.

In addition to those mentioned above, here are a few more examples of conditions that are significant:

Anemia

Heart disease

Heart murmur, or any other
   heart irregularity

HIV

Herpes

Multiple sclerosis

Nerve paralysis

Cancer of any form

Diabetes

Gingivitis (gum or periodontal
   disease)

Hemophilia

Kleptomania (just making sure
   you're paying attention)

Epilepsy

Gulf War syndrome

Alcohol or other addictions

Vertigo
Sexual dysfunction
Paraplegia or quadriplegia
Sleep apnea
Vision or hearing loss
Glaucoma
Parkinson's disease
Amputation

Liver disease
Post-traumatic stress disorder
Dementia or frequent memory
  loss (for example, can't recall
  name of close friend or
  relative)
Multicythemia veragis (just
  kidding)

Here are some that are probably not significant:

Astigmatism
Dental cavities
Sore lower back after shoveling
  heavy snow
Rosacea
Varicose veins
Toenail fungus infection or
  athlete's foot
Forgetfulness (for example,
  can't remember where keys are,
  or where you were when
  Luke and Laura married on
  General Hospital)

Sunburn prone or can't tan
Insomnia before job interviews
  or court sentencings
Cat allergy
Hangover
Irritability
Disorganization
C-SPAN addiction
Turkey neck
Repeatedly date or marry losers

Now list your *past* significant ailments and conditions in the next section, noting when you were diagnosed and what happened. Then list all the details about the medications you're taking (*all* pills or tablets or anything that you regularly

Checklist: We Ask, You Answer

For any condition or ailment you include on your list that you're still dealing with, write down and be prepared to tell the doc the following:

- ☐ What caused this?
- ☐ When was it diagnosed?
- ☐ How are you treating it?
- ☐ Has it gotten better or worse?
- ☐ When did it first begin to noticeably improve or worsen?
- ☐ What makes it better?
- ☐ What makes it worse?

ingest, inject, insert, or otherwise consume regularly, whether it's prescription or over-the-counter (OTC) drugs, herbal supplements, vitamins, etc.). We'll say this again, but in addition to having this form handy when you see your doctor (in your pocket or the office file cabinet), always bring the actual bottles of all those medicinal consumables, too. It's important.

Don't Know Much about Genealogy

On pages 52 and 53, you'll also find the Smart Patient Family Tree. Flip to it and sharpen a pencil. This Smart Patient Family

Mom

Tree is designed to bring joy (and longevity) to your life. The solid lines sprouting outward from you to your siblings, and downward to your parents, aunts and uncles, and grandparents represent *blood-relative connections* (not by marriage). You'll notice a dashed line going to your spouse, which represents a non–blood relationship. The reason you need to include your spouse is that he or she lives with you (at least we hope so). That means you share the same environmental exposures and, likely, similar risks. You serve as each other's personal coalmine canary. One of you may get nauseous from the toxic waste buried under your house years before the other one.

Dad

(Just kidding! You'd likely be afflicted simultaneously.) Also, even though you don't share DNA (at least not on most school nights, anyway), your spouse influences your health far more than your aunt Sadie in Perth Amboy. Auntie may have a cholesterol count that would bring a Guinness World Records rep to her door, but she isn't filling your day-to-day life with cigarette smoke, bacon, Pabst Blue Ribbon, and lost-sock arguments. The only thing worse for your health and longevity than having a spouse is *not* having one, in fact. No one likes being nagged, but being nagged into eating broccoli pays dividends.

Start filling out the Smart Patient Family Tree by adding your spouse's info, if you have one. You'll notice that the tree reaches only to your grandparents, not back to your Viking ancestors like some other family trees you may have seen. Why? Of course you recall the genetic Mendel grid from biology class, and how a fruit fly's ability to pass his tiny wings to his great-grandson was so genetically diluted, it was practically nil. Alas, the apple never falls far from the tree, but the fruit fly must at least be in the orchard—that is, at least as genetically close as a grandparent—before you go blaming him for any shortcomings.

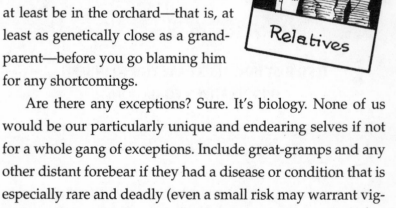

Relatives

Are there any exceptions? Sure. It's biology. None of us would be our particularly unique and endearing selves if not for a whole gang of exceptions. Include great-gramps and any other distant forebear if they had a disease or condition that is especially rare and deadly (even a small risk may warrant vigilance or gene testing). For example, Baron von Munchausen VI is still at extreme risk, but he knows that.

Thicken your family tree with all the info you know

offhand. You want to record each relative's birth date and (if applicable) death date, the jobs they performed (as certain occupations can strongly affect health), and—most important—any diseases they had that may have a genetic link. Your doctor can clarify this if you aren't certain about the disease or if it was never diagnosed. Just list the symptoms the person had (memory loss, for example). While you're at it, you might as well jot down any other interesting tidbits in case the kids get curious about their roots one day. If you're like most people, it'll be about 14 percent complete when your brain is tapped. You'll need to do some investigating, Columbo style (Remember? Smart cop?), so see the checklist (on page 54) for the family interrogation protocol.

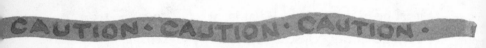

CAUTION • CAUTION • CAUTION •

TEST: JUST HOW LIKELY ARE YOU TO INHERIT THIS RELATIVE'S CONDITION?

To better assess your risk, answer these questions for each relative who has (or had) a disease that might be genetically transmissible to you:

Y / N **Is this an immediate, full-blood relative?** Circle yes if it is your mother or father or a sibling (if a stepsibling, circle no)

Y / N **Did this relative get the disease with a suspected genetic link *before* age sixty-five?**

Y / N **Did this relative die from this disease before age sixty-five?**

Y / N   **Was this disease likely caused by a genetic link, and not caused by environmental or lifestyle factors?** (If the relative was a heavy smoker, a heavy drinker, or had a toxic or hazardous exposure at work, and these likely caused or contributed to the disease, circle no)

Y / N   **Is there at least one other blood relative who also has or had any of these same diseases?**

Y / N   **Do you look like this relative, either inside or out?** Meaning, do you have the same body type, same cholesterol problem, same bad temper, etc.?

If you circled one or two Ys, you may be at risk for inheriting this condition, so monitor it with your doctor. You circled three or more Ys? You're likely at very high risk of inheriting the disease, so keep a watchful eye on it.

Hopefully, you won't have to interrogate more than a handful of relatives in the above manner. If you hail from a litter of fourteen and have more aunts than a cartoon picnic, however, just remember to keep your radar sharp for two factors: serious illness or death before age sixty-five, and potentially fatal conditions. Either can be more important than how close you and your relative are in the bloodline. For example, your uncle's pancreatic cancer at age fifty-three would likely be more alarming to us than your mother's heart fibrillations at age seventy. At a bare minimum, you need to know why your parents and grandparents died, if they're now gone. And your bottom-line question to your doctor is always the same: If there's a genetic link associated with this condition, how can I prevent it?

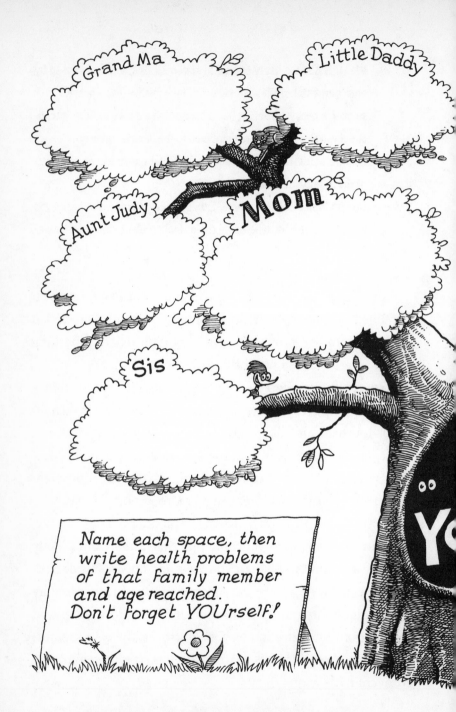

The Smart Patient Family Tree

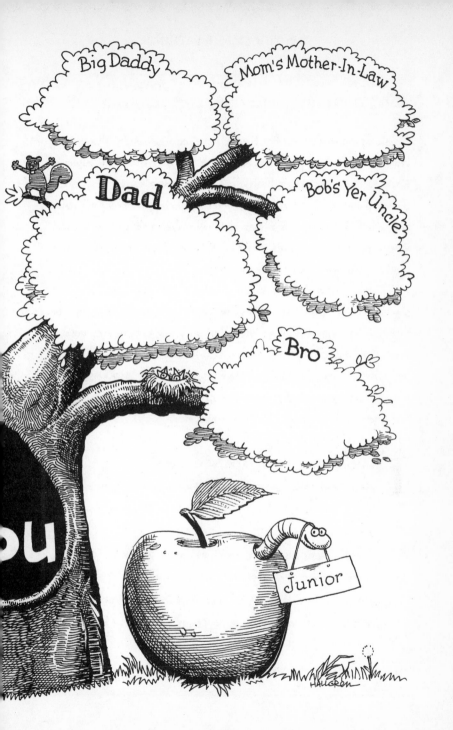

Checklist: Gastritis, Aunt Gertrude?

Shaking down family for health details needn't always be a horribly awkward task. Remember that half will always talk about the other half, so go the gossip route if easier. If you want to be direct, just grab your reporter's pad and pen, dial the phone or meet the relative at the early-bird diner, and repeat this checklist (feel free to ad-lib). You might consider an opener like this:

"Hello, [relative]. I know you haven't heard from me since [year], but I'm putting my family health history together to see if I'm at risk for anything genetic, and I thought you could tell me a few things I just can't find anywhere else. [Another relative he or she dislikes] said you probably wouldn't help me or wouldn't be able to remember, but I thought I'd try anyway."

☐ When were you born? (Or "Who was the first president you remember?" if the relative won't say. If it's Franklin Delano Roosevelt, ask if he or she voted for him.)

☐ Have you been diagnosed with any diseases? When?

☐ What kind of treatment did you get?

☐ Any cancers? Diabetes? Heart problems? High blood pressure? Do you take any drugs (not those kind) or supplements? If so, why?

☐ Any surgeries? When, and for what?

- ☐ Ever have a bout of depression, anxiety, or other emotional health problems? (Ask relative this family member dislikes for immediate answer.)
- ☐ Any miscarriages, stillbirths, or infant deaths?
- ☐ Any heart attacks or strokes? (Pretend you suddenly remember and ask if the flowers made it.)
- ☐ How's your hearing? (Whispered.)
- ☐ Do you or did you smoke or drink?
- ☐ What jobs did you have?
- ☐ Still lead in the pencil?
- ☐ Has your memory deteriorated? Do you still remember my name?
- ☐ So, that thing growing on [another relative]—is that skin cancer or what?

A Day in Your Life

Woke up, fell out of bed . . .

Dragged a comb across your head. Then you found your way downstairs and dra . . . all right, you get it. One of the most time-intensive but valuable parts of your health profile is to get a detailed description of your typical day. We start by asking what time you generally wake up in the morning (and how, whether you're roused by dawn's gentle light, a rooster,

Home, Hazardous Home

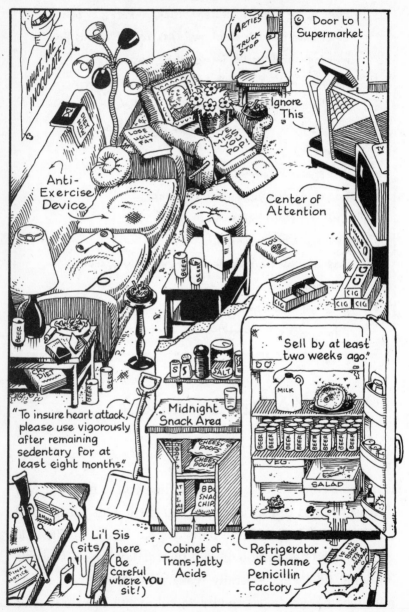

an amorous mate, a lapping cat, morning smoker's cough, and so on) and how refreshed you typically feel. Next we ask about morning chores, the length and stress of the work commute, the first task (or taskmaster) to greet you at the office, and the sordid toils and pleasures of the entire A.M. journey. Then we discuss your typical lunch. You can see why this takes a while. But it's valuable in getting a full picture of your life and an accurate depiction of the suspects and scenes that affect your health, as demonstrated in these illustrations. Hopefully, this home setting won't look too much like yours.

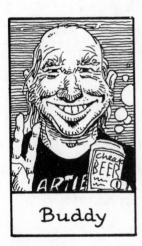

Buddy

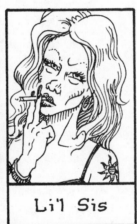

Li'l Sis

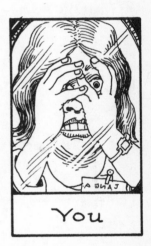

You

We Double Trouble

We know you bend the truth a little when telling us the good and bad you do to yourself. That's why we at least double, up or down, the most fudged claims. For example:

CAUTION · CAUTION · CAUTION ·

PATIENT SAYS	WE HEAR
I have two drinks a day.	I might drink a case a week.
I exercise about twice a week.	I rarely exercise.
I smoke a few cigarettes a day.	I'm a pack-a-day-er.
I smoked for five years.	I smoked for ten years and off and on for a few more.
My job is stressful.	This job's going to give me a coronary if I don't quit or learn how to deal with it.
I hardly ever have unsafe sex.	I use condoms about half the time.
I get short of breath if I run.	Five porch steps leave me gasping.
I eat about two hamburgers a week.	I eat cheeseburgers most of the other days.
I forget to take my medication about once a week.	I remember to take my medication about twice a week.
I'll follow up with you; I won't forget.	I'll stop back in when the kids are grown.

The Adopted Plan

Logging your genetic propensities is enough of a job when you have your blood relatives close at hand or accessible in your address book. But what if you're adopted? Or if you've adopted a child? Thousands face this hurdle each year in compiling a health history. Luckily, it's becoming a bit less difficult to get the information you need.

There's a trend in domestic adoptions toward openness—in other words, the adoptee, birth parent (one or both), and adoptive family all have a degree of contact with one another and share relevant information, including health histories. Recent laws have helped unseal files too. Of course, there are still many adoptees and adoptive parents who have no such contact or any records whatsoever, for a host of different reasons, and have come up empty even after checking with the adoption agency (always the first place to contact on this mission). In this case, they should contact their state Department of Health and Human Services to see if any birth records exist, and also examine the various registries that attempt to link birth families and adopted persons. A great all-around source is the government's National Adoption Information Clearinghouse Web site at **naic.acf.hhs.gov.** You can search by state for info and availability of records. Remember that there's no need for a tearful, emotional reunion if that's not wanted: these registries often connect adoptees and birth parents for the sole purpose of gathering health information.

What about international adoptions? Some countries are

TIP: HAVE A TATTLE PLAN

Bring your spouse to your doctor's appointment when you're giving your health history; there are a lot of questions that only he or she can answer (how many times an hour do you stop breathing while asleep?). But, please, before coming in to the office together, make sure you discuss which fibs you're going to tell the doctor. Why? Because when you tell us that you rarely tear into the Pringles after 8:00 P.M. or that you've been taking your cholesterol-lowering drugs with the discipline of a marine, your spouse will shoot you—or us—an involuntary look that communicates something close to *Are you kidding me?* We never miss it. And, hey, sometimes your spouse *wants* to blow your cover. It's called love—why do you think she booked the appointment?

If you try to snow us, remember that we might try to trip you up by asking about specific dates. As in when you last did something. For example, we'll ask you if you're fit enough to climb three flights of stairs. You'll say yes, unless you're older than eighty-five or bedbound. Then we'll ask, "When was the *last time* you climbed three flights of stairs?" You'll think, and start to say, "Maybe a month, or . . ." and your spouse will shoot that never-fails look. The one that says, *You haven't climbed three flights of stairs since we voted for Ike.*

How embarrassing.

So please, rehearse beforehand.

just beginning to open their records, and the adoption agency and country consulate's office can be a starting point for investigation.

A Ghoulish Notion?

If your parents will consent to it, consider having an autopsy performed on them when they die. Few autopsies are done today as compared with decades ago, as it's rarely thought necessary when a cause of death is clear, such as a heart attack. But there's much value in knowing if your eighty-two-year-old father had undiagnosed prostate cancer that had been advancing since his fifties, or heart disease, even though it was a stroke that did him in. This is especially useful if the death was due to an accident, of course. Reassure your living parent that this doesn't mean foul play is suspected, or that the body will be shipped to a *CSI* soundstage, or that there can't be an open casket.

CLICK ACCESS TO YOUR HEALTH INFO

There are several Web sites that allow you to store your health records online, so you, your doctor, or any person given permission can tap them on the Internet, from any location. Some are free, and others have monthly fees that range from $30 to $80. To check out a few examples, click into the Web sites at **www.ihealth record.org, www.personalhealthkey.com, healthmanager.web md.com,** and the Joint Commission Resources' own **www.jcrinc .com.** We'll update this list at the personal-health site at **www .realage.com.** Each site has security safeguards to protect the confidentiality of your info. Aside from the convenience factor, using these sites could make it easier to you keep your files current, because you'll have a one-stop, central place to update your info.

2

Finding Dr. Right

How to Find That Gem of a Doctor
Who'll Make Your Life Easier—and Longer

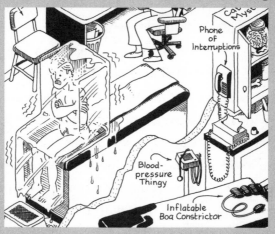

One of the most important decisions you will ever make—and one you'll likely make more than once—is choosing your doctor. As the owner of a wondrous commodity (your body), you always have supreme rule, but your doctor is the get-it-done person. Consider your doc to be the head coach of your football team, the floor manager of your Hollywood restaurant, the captain of your ocean liner. Choose wisely, and you could rest easy for many years to come, knowing that your sentinel is on the job, on the ball, and taking care of the duties you need done. Pick an incompetent boob who talks a good game, or even a well-respected professional who is hopelessly overbooked and can't find the time to squeeze you in, and your boat may sink.

We've seen it happen. And we've been called in on salvage operations.

A Smart Patient will pick his or her doctor wisely. Sometimes, picking your doctor wisely means walking out of a doc's office if he or she isn't the best choice for you, or understanding if we give you a referral to a trusted colleague. A Smart Doctor chooses his or her patients wisely too. Today there are so many advanced subspecialties of medicine, and so many physicians who have developed expertise in particular specialties while still operating as primary-care physicians, that matching the right patient with the right doctor is a far more complex—but rewarding—mission than it was just a few decades ago.

Marcus Welby (whom we will continue to abuse, with our apologies to the late Robert Young) seemed to handle the limitless gamut of his patients with equal ease, graciousness, and expertise. Today, if he attempted to keep the same philosophy, he wouldn't find enough hours in the week to give half of those patients cutting-edge care. He'd be a likable, dangerously ineffectual physician to many of his patients—so affable and likable that many wouldn't know that he was unqualified to treat them until something bad happened. Until, say, that beauty mark he repeatedly told you not to worry about turned out to be melanoma, because while he might be a great internist, he's not a dermatologist.

You, however, won't run into these problems. Because you're going to choose—or requalify and, if necessary, replace—your physician with an insider's eye, using the criteria that will ensure he or she is the absolute best primary-care doctor (PCD) for you. You need the facts. So we'll give you the questions to ask while you're channeling Joe Friday (remember, you just want the facts, ma'am).

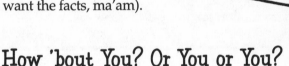

Sgt. Joe Friday

How 'bout You? Or You or You?

There's a shortage of physicians in the United States, and medical schools aren't pumping out numbers to match the increase in population (though women now make up the slight majority of graduates, so not all of the news is dismal). Still, we have more than 700,000 doctors, and if you open your insurance plan's in-network directory, you'll see a bevy of white coats in your area. They all have different backgrounds, different approaches to care, different specialties, and different levels of skill. How can you pick the right one without visiting at least twenty-nine or becoming frustrated and just randomly plunk-

TIP: CARRY ON

If the doctor doesn't accept your insurance, but he or she is really your top choice, don't give up. Call the insurer and ask if it would consider adding this doctor to its list. If the company won't, ask why. Sometimes, if even just a few patients call and ask an insurer to add a doctor, it will. Likewise, ask your doctor if you could convince him or her to begin accepting your insurer. And every year when you renew your health insurance (a lovely period in November called *open enrollment* by most employers), call your doctor and make sure he or she intends to keep accepting this insurance plan. When doctors are deciding which insurance carriers we'll work with, we can be swayed by just a few small factors. If dropping a plan will create big problems for two or three regular and Smart Patients, that can carry weight. So speak up.

ing your finger down on the page? Further, what if none of them is the best choice, and you'd be better off paying more for a physician who isn't on that list? Paying *much* more, that is. It can make you want to drink.

Before you reach for the bottle, though, let's tackle it together.

Find Your PCD ASAP

Although the tips we're giving you will work in qualifying any doctor—from a cardiologist to a podiatrist to an internist;

most any-*ist*, in fact—the doctor we're talking about here is your primary-care physician. Or the head football coach that we referred to earlier. If your health insurance is a health maintenance organization (HMO) or other managed-care plan, you know all too well what a primary-care physician is. Such plans most often require you to have one on record. This main doctor tends to your everyday health care needs and is often the "gate-keeper" in referring you to other physicians when you need a specialist, such as a dermatologist or a psychiatrist or a special surgeon.

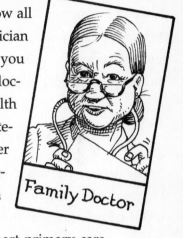

Family Doctor

As a Smart Patient choosing a smart primary-care doc, you're really looking for a physician who's smart with referrals and has connections with the best specialists in your part of the country.

Primary-care physicians typically include:

Family practitioners, who treat patients of all ages

General practitioners, who may treat children, adults, or both

Internists, who treat adults

Doctors of osteopathic medicine (DOs)

Obstetricians/gynecologists, who treat women

Pediatricians, who treat infants, children and teenagers

Your primary physician will probably be the one you see the most often, and he or she should know your complete medical history, which you handily completed in the last chapter (or will soon, right?). You're also likely to have the closest relationship with your primary-care physician, so it's critical to feel comfortable with this doctor and to have confidence in him or her. If you don't, you'll probably skip routine preventive-care visits and other appointments that aren't absolutely necessary to keep you getting around on two feet, and that's asking for trouble.

A-Hunting We Will Go

People love to exchange horror stories about doctors' offices, like the ones shown on page 69.

Of course, the first thing you'll do when searching for a doctor—or a roofer, or plumber, or hairstylist—is ask your friends, neighbors, and coworkers for a referral. If you're lucky enough to have a relative or friend who works in health care (don't forget paramedics and emergency medical technicians, or EMTs), make a beeline for him, of course. Bring coffee cake. If your family is devoid of any health care connection, soliciting opinions on people's primary-care doctors can lead to great referrals, but they might be short on substance. "Dr. Todd is *wonderful!*" Aunt Frieda will say, looking at the heavens in rapture. As a starting point, this is a great way to begin. But in considering that Aunt Frieda also gave your phone number to that loon on the bus so you two could date, she might not be the best authority on who you should trust with your life.

Don't Go Doctor's Office

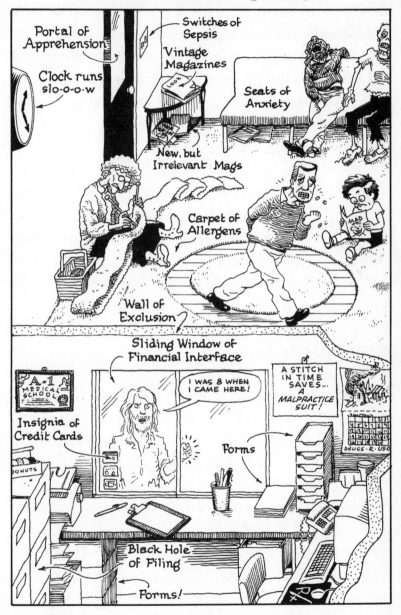

After combing your cadre of friends and loved ones, you can subject any emergent candidates to higher scrutiny. But in all likelihood, you'll be starting from scratch, perhaps with only the list of physicians in your managed-care directory. If you don't have this directory, ask your employer's human-resources department for a copy or call the insurer directly; these physician lists are usually available online, too.

To find Dr. Right, follow these steps.

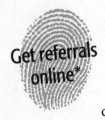

Get referrals online*

The Internet is the fastest, easiest modern medium for finding the needle-in-a-haystack doctor who's a perfect match for you. These sites are good choices, though some cater to certain specialties. Finding a particular doctor listed on two or more is a good sign.

American Medical Association

www.ama-assn.org

The American Medical Association's Web site includes stories about medical issues and news and lets you search for doctors by name or medical specialty. It also has a "Group Practice Locator," which lets you search for practice groups by state.

---

* We won't bother saying "If you have Internet access . . . ," because obviously, it's absolutely critical for being a Smart Patient and, to a growing degree every day, remaining a part of this wacky evolving thing we call human society. Trying to become a Smart Patient without having Internet access would be akin to trying to assemble a jigsaw puzzle while wearing a blindfold. You can get online free at any library if you don't have a computer at home.

American Board of Medical Specialties
www.abms.org

This site lets you determine whether a doctor is board certified and search for board-certified physicians.

American College of Physicians
www.acponline.org

The American College of Physicians' Web site provides good information about its physician members and advocacy programs.

American College of Surgeons
www.facs.org

The American College of Surgeons' Web site has a special section for patients to help them choose qualified surgeons. It also includes answers to patients' frequently asked questions about operations, including getting a second opinion and giving your informed consent.

Diabetes Physician Recognition Program
www.ncqa.org/dprp

This site was developed by the National Committee for Quality Assurance (NCQA) and the American Diabetes Association (ADA) to recognize physicians who demonstrate high-quality care for patients with diabetes.

Family Doctor
www.familydoctor.org

This site, sponsored by the American Association of Family Physicians (AAFP), includes more than two hundred clinically reviewed articles on health topics for men, women, and children. You can also search for physicians who are members of the AAFP by zip code.

Healthfinder
www.healthfinder.gov

This health-library search engine was developed by the U.S. Department of Health and Human Services and allows users to search for information about different health topics and drugs, and provides a directory of doctors, dentists, and hospitals; it also provides links to health organizations and other resources.

Heart/Stroke Recognition Program
www.ncqa.org/hsrp

This site, developed by NCQA and the American Heart Association/American Stroke Association (AHA/ASA), recognizes physicians who demonstrate high-quality care for patients who have had a stroke or have cardiac conditions.

Medline Plus
www.medlineplus.gov

This site is sponsored by the U.S. National Library of Medicine (NLM) and the National Institutes of Health (NIH) and includes current health news, drug information, a medical encyclopedia, and resources for finding doctors, dentists, and hospitals.

Call a medical society for referrals Flip to appendix 3, Resources, and find the list entitled "Find a Board-Certified Doctor." The American Board of Medical Specialties (ABMS) recognizes twenty-four areas of medical specialty, including anesthesiology, cardiology, internal medicine, and pediatrics. Most of these subgroups will refer you to physicians on their list in your area. Does that mean you can simply pick one of these names and be assured of having the best doctor? No. But you can be assured that these doctors have passed muster with somebody else besides Aunt Frieda. A board-certified doctor has passed exams in a certain specialty, so it's evidence of skill. Personally, we wouldn't go to a doctor who wasn't board certified, and it's one of the first things we'll investigate when finding a doctor or specialist for our family members. But to be fair, it's optional to become certified, and not all doctors choose to do it, so we're sure there are some excellent doctors who aren't board certified. We just wouldn't take our kids to them or let them operate on us. Other doctors may be listed as *board eligible*, which means they haven't taken the exam yet, or they failed it. To quickly find out if a doctor you're seeing or considering is board certified, call the American Board of Medical Specialties at 866-275-2267 or click on **www.abms.org.**

Grill the ER nurse manager at the best local hospital

A nearby trusted hospital would be best. A nurse in the intensive-care unit is also a good choice, if you have the occasion to get in there. ERs are a little more accessible than ICUs if you're on a fact-finding mission. These registered nurses get a battlefield view of doctors at their best and worst. They know who's sharp, who's respected, who stays on top of things, who sees their patients and knows what they are doing in the ER, who uses the best consultants, and who guesses correctly 80 percent of the time. They also know which doctors are indecisive, which ones get second-guessed, which ones tend to get their tests delayed, which ones guess correctly 40 percent of the time, and which ones are unusually slow in answering pages. If a doctor doesn't have privileges at the best local hospital, that's an argument to look for a different doctor.

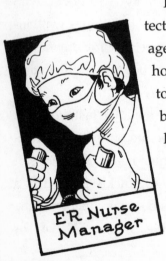

ER Nurse Manager

How can you go about this bit of detective work to find that ER nurse manager? Visiting a friend or relative in the hospital provides a good opportunity to swing into the unit. If all hell isn't breaking loose there and the nurses have a few relatively quiet minutes (midmorning on a weekday is usually best), you'll have a chance to politely approach one and make your inquiry. A good script? "I have to choose a new doctor who has privileges at this hospital, most ideally one who is particularly good at treating patients with diabetes [or the condition that concerns you]. I've been doing a lot of research, and I realize all the physicians here are great, but I wanted to just ask you—in knowing what you know—which specific doctors you might take a closer look at if you were in my position."

If you get the wrong nurse, you won't get a helpful answer. If you get the right one, and you've presented yourself well, you'll get at least one name and a reason. Just keep in mind that these nurses are seeing aspects of medical care that you're not, and they may choose a particular doctor for reasons that may not wholly jibe with your own preferences. An example? A nurse might say, "Well, to be honest, Dr. So-and-So is a complete jerk, and everybody hates him, but if you're in serious trouble there's nobody better." People being mixed bags, endorsements like this aren't unusual in medicine. The nurse may be able to help with a quick introduction if things are unusually quiet. Having a cup of coffee with her couldn't hurt.

Dr. Knowitall

If you wangle the opportunity to ask this question of an ER doctor, or a critical-care doctor who works in the intensive-care unit, don't pass it up. They work directly with primary-care doctors.

The above tactics will generate more than a few likely candidates. Once you have this list of potential primary-care physicians, investigate each one by looking him up on the Internet, and by calling his office and asking the questions in the following checklist.

A Ploy Named Sue

What about malpractice claims? Finding out if a doctor has been sued for botched practicing is certainly a legitimate factor in qualifying him or her, as long as the info is put into context. To find out if any malpractice lawsuits have been filed against a physician, call the county clerk's office where he or she practices, as well as the state medical-licensing board and the state insurance department. (You can ask the latter if any claims are on record for the doctor.) You can also check your doctor's record on Web sites such as **www.docboard.org.** Just remember that it's common for doctors to be sued, and many cases are dismissed or won by physicians, so the fact that a doctor has been sued for malpractice isn't necessarily a damning sign. However, if the doctor has been sued several times in the last few years, and many of those suits have been settled or resulted in large awards to patients, we as doctors would see that as a warning sign to move on. Lightning can indeed strike in the same spot twice, but four or five times is a little troubling.

Good Questions, Good Answers

If a doctor looks like a promising choice, call the office and do some detective work.

YOU ASK: Is the doctor accepting new patients?

GOOD ANSWER: "Yes." Or "Possibly." Or "Not right now." You want a busy physician with plenty of patients. Just as you'd rather order pasta in a crowded restaurant instead of one that's bone empty. "No" really means, "Get to know the office manager and be persistent, and you'll get in within a few weeks or months."

SHAKY ANSWER: "You bet. He hasn't seen anyone all week, and, boy, is he bored."

YOU ASK: Is this doctor working primarily in management?

GOOD ANSWER: "No, she only sees patients," or "Yes, but she sees patients at least one day a week."

SHAKY ANSWER: "Yes, and she only sees patients when she can." A physician who's managing the careers of ninety people might have a difficult time making your care her top priority. Patients rarely consider this when they demand to have the "chief" be their primary-care doc. Many managing docs were great practicing doctors, and many still are— but if they don't see patients regularly, at least one day a week, you may be exchanging status for the best care.

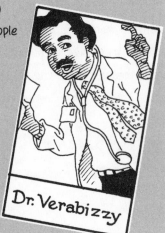

Dr. Verabizzy

YOU ASK: Where did the doctor study and do her residency?

GOOD ANSWER: An accredited medical school and residency program in the United States. Click on the AMA's DoctorFinder to check out both at www.ama-assn.org/aps.

SHAKY ANSWER: An unaccredited school, or a foreign medical school. Many foreign medical schools are great, and some are superior to many U.S. schools, but standards vary widely. Investigate the doctor's medical school if it's on foreign shores.

YOU ASK: Which types of patients does the doctor usually see?

GOOD ANSWER: People who seem fairly similar to you with similar health issues.

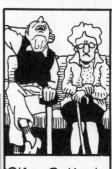

Other Patients

SHAKY ANSWER: People who don't seem to have any similarities to you (for example, would you go to a pediatrician if you were twenty-nine?).

YOU ASK: What insurance plan do you accept?

 GOOD ANSWER: Yours.

SHAKY ANSWER: Not yours. See the tip "Carry On" on page 66.

YOU ASK: Where does the doctor have hospital privileges? (Meaning, at which hospital is he or she allowed to treat patients?)

GOOD ANSWER: A Joint Commission accredited hospital. Or an accredited hospital that excels in treating certain conditions, specifically yours. Having privileges at a big teaching hospital is a good sign, too. See chapter 5 for more on this.

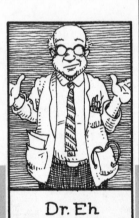

Dr. Eh

SHAKY ANSWER: None, or a hospital not accredited by the Joint Commission, or only at the smallest one in a fifty-mile radius.

YOU ASK: Who typically cares for the doctor's patients at the office or the hospital when she's out?

GOOD ANSWER: A specific doctor who has equally strong credentials and training. Or specialists that this doctor will keep in touch with daily. Or, in the hospital, a hospitalist. See the sidebar "A Funny Word for a Good Doctor" on page 86.

SHAKY ANSWER: It varies from day to day.

YOU ASK: Would the doctor covering for her have complete access to all of my medical records?

GOOD ANSWER: Yes.

SHAKY ANSWER: No.

YOU ASK: In the office, does the doctor practice alone or with other physicians?

GOOD ANSWER: With other physicians who have equally strong credentials and training.

SHAKY ANSWER: Alone, unless you live in a rural area where that's the norm.

YOU ASK: Is the doctor board certified by an American Board of Medical Specialties (ABMS) Program?

GOOD ANSWER: Yes. The board certifications from the ABMS have to be earned the old-fashioned way: by passing tough exams. To check out the physician, look him or her up on www.abms.org.

SHAKY ANSWER: No. Or yes, but in a specialty that is not of concern to you given your specific needs.

YOU ASK: How long has the doctor been board certified?

GOOD ANSWER: Longer than three years.

SHAKY ANSWER: Less than three years.

YOU ASK: Is the doctor especially qualified to treat patients with your condition?

GOOD ANSWER: Yes, because she acquired specific training or has specific certification. The office administrator or office assistant can usually tell you this.

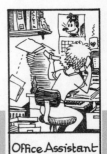

Office Assistant

SHAKY ANSWER: No. Or yes, she'd be fine because she sees all types of patients. But no evidence is given as to why the doctor is specially qualified to meet your needs.

YOU ASK: Who else would she recommend if she couldn't take me on as a patient?

GOOD ANSWER (after actually speaking with the doctor): "She would recommend [specific doctor with equally strong or better training], because of [a specific reason]."

SHAKY ANSWER: Her relative or friend, who isn't specially qualified to treat you. Or no one special, check your HMO directory.

YOU ASK: Do other doctors use this physician for their own care?

GOOD ANSWER: Yes. The office manager is also a good source for this.

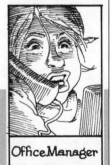

OfficeManager

SHAKY ANSWER: No, or very few.

Are You Paging Old Dr. Young or Young Dr. Young?

How old should your physician be? That's a personal preference. Age is never a driving factor, but it does bring in a couple of considerations in picking a primary-care doctor. An advantage to choosing one who's roughly your age or a little younger? You two can age together. Because you ideally want to build a long relationship with this doctor, picking a fantastic physician who's considering retirement in a couple years might not be the best choice. (Although this physician might be the specialist you need to see after choosing another primary-care doctor.) Naturally, you'll be lucky to keep one physician your whole life; most people move several times, and you need a primary-care doctor who is close enough to visit without buying a plane ticket. But give it the best odds possible. Having a doctor who knows you well is a huge advantage.

Another consideration is whether your doctor keeps up with cutting-edge advancements in medicine. Older doctors bring more experience to your care, but if their subscription to the *Journal of the American Medical Association (JAMA)* lapsed in 1988, that could be a problem. Sure, this is an ageist stereotype, and some of the older docs are far more on the ball than the young bucks. Just as you wouldn't necessarily want a wet-eared doctor overseeing your health, entrusting it to Mr. Magoo might not be a hot idea, either.

YOU DID WHAT?

You know your doctor went to college and then did another four-year stint in medical school, at minimum. If he didn't, that framed degree came from the local print shop. Below is a translation of some other terms you'll hear when inquiring about a doctor's background.

* **Internship:** the first year of training following medical school. This is now often called the first year of residency.
* **Residency:** a period of three to seven years of specialty training after medical school.
* **Board certification:** means that a doctor has passed exams given by the American Board of Medical Specialties in one or more of twenty-four specialties.
* **Licensure:** the legal permission to practice medicine in a particular area, granted by a state or territory after a physician passes an exam.

A FUNNY WORD FOR A GOOD DOCTOR

The hospitalist. Sounds like a Sylvester Stallone movie. Actually it's a term for a doctor you ought to know. Hospitalists are doctors who work only (guess where?) in hospitals and are especially trained to care for patients who are sicker and require more treatment than those your primary-care doctor sees in the office. Whenever you're in the hospital, there's a good chance that you'll have one of these physicians caring for you as your full-time in-hospital doctor or covering for your primary doctor. When you're shopping for a primary-care doctor, these doctors are one of the best info sources. Don't fail to question one if you're visiting a relative or friend in the hospital; in fact, it's a good excuse to visit someone. Your kid's school janitor will never forget that his hernia operation meant so much to you.

It's a Date

You've selected a doctor? It's time for an audition, then. Schedule a visit. You're better off meeting a new physician for a simple checkup when there's nothing seriously wrong. This will give you a stress-free chance to appraise the doctor and the office employees. Also, if you're not a morning person, try to repent. Whenever you book a doctor's appointment, always try to be one of the first appointments of the day. At that time, things haven't had a chance to become hopelessly backed up, as they typically have by the fifteenth appointment. Why? Most doctors schedule appointments in fifteen-minute segments, and studies show that the average appointment lasts between eighteen and twenty minutes. Mix in late patients, no-shows, and a host of other time wasters, and you'll see why you've always spent more time in the waiting room than talking to the doctor. And spending an afternoon chilling out in the waiting room or waiting for the doctor in the examination room could make you feel a lot like the patient shown in the next illustration. If you have a lot to discuss, tell the office receptionist, so he or she can help. You might also consider asking if you can book two segments. You will probably have to pay for both, depending on your doctor (and your health insurer may not cover the second appointment), and your insurance company, but some patients occasionally do this in special circumstances when they really don't want to risk feeling rushed.

A tip: befriend the office nurses and the administrators. They can make your life very pleasant and convenient in dealing with your doctor, so show them love at every visit. Learn their names. Their hometowns. Bring small gifts. Dip strawberries in dark chocolate. Have your child draw a picture for them. Write a thank-you note. It'll pay dividends.

Finally, whether it's your first visit with a physician or you've been seeing the doctor for decades, one way to save time (and that means saving money) is to have everything that could possibly be useful in your hand or in the file cabinet in the doctor's back office. Use the checklist on page 90 to make sure you're all set.

Edgy Examination Room

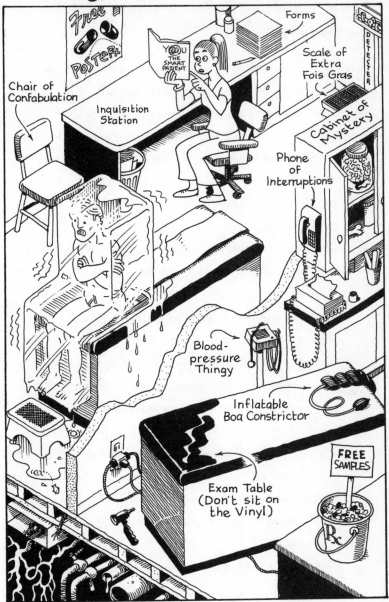

Checklist: The Smart Patient Motto: Be Prepared

Okay, we cribbed that from the Boy Scouts, but it gets to the heart of it. Before your appointment with the doctor, be certain you have everything you need. Even if your visit is a routine checkup, hit this checklist before any doctor's appointment to be through and avoid missing anything:

☐ Do I have my filled-out health profile to take to the appointment?

☐ What questions do I have for the doctor about my health profile? Write these down.

☐ What other documents or items do I need to bring to the appointment (such as X-rays, pathology reports, or other medical records)?

☐ Do I need to have any other physicians send my prior medical records to the new doctor's office?

☐ Do I have all of my insurance information handy?

☐ In addition to my written medication list, do I have the actual bottles and containers of every single prescription medication, over-the-counter drug, herbal supplement, vitamin, and anything else I take regularly all bundled neatly to bring to the appointment?

☐ Who do I want to come with me to the appointment?

☐ Do I need to do anything special (such as fast for twelve hours for a blood glucose test, for example) before the appointment?

☐ Do I have my tape recorder, with a blank tape and fresh batteries?

☐ Which specific questions do I want answered at this appointment? Write these down. You may have several, but these four are definitely among them:

    ☐ How is my health overall?

    ☐ Are you concerned about any aspect of my health? Which one(s) and why?

    ☐ Are there any tests I should have based on my age or for other reasons?

    ☐ Do you have any recommendations about lifestyle modifications I should make (such as exercising, quitting smoking, or changing my diet and in what specific ways)?

What's a-Matter You?

You've booked the appointment? Great. The first thing any doctor will ask you—thus the first thing you need to prepare a cogent answer to—is "What's wrong with you?" We may phrase this question as "What brings you here?" or "What can I do you for?," but you'll know what we really mean. By the way, if we ask, "What brings you here today?" and you reply, "Oh, nothing in particular," or, "Several different things," we may consider jumping out the window. We translate these responses as "I'm going to give you vague symptoms and troubles while going off on tangents, and then expect you to give me a specific treatment."

If you're there to check us out as a potential primary-care doctor, tell us. Give us the stuff you filled out in chapter 1 and watch how we perform. If you want to discuss a particular problem, like your weight, or headaches, be prepared with some specifics. A Smart Patient describes medical problems straightforwardly in as much detail as possible—without breaking into a story about how Uncle Smitty had the same problem, except it was in the other leg.

How much detail is enough? If you say you're having headaches, *where* do you experience the pain? Is it in the front of your head, at your temples, at the base of your skull, or throughout your entire head? *What* kind of pain is it: a dull throbbing, a sharp piercing, or a constant ache? *How* severe is the pain? *When* does it occur and how often? *When* did the headaches start? Have you been able to do anything to make the pain better? *What* makes it worse? Does it wake you at night or keep you from sleeping? The more detail you can provide, the better. In fact, more than 80 percent of health problems can be diagnosed by the information the patient provides his or her doctor.

Restated, be ready to talk to your doctor about these factors for any problem you have:

Cause—have you noticed what, if anything, triggers the symptoms?

Severity—how bad is the pain or symptom? We'll often ask you to rate the pain on a scale of one to ten, with one being no pain and ten being the worst pain you can imagine. Everyone always gives a number *and a half,* as in six and a half. Six or seven would do.

Previous or current treatments—have you tried any medications, dietary changes, or other treatments? Have they made a difference in your symptoms?

Checklist: This Is a Test

Your doctor wants you to have an MRI (magnetic resonance imaging), or a CT (computed tomography) scan, or some other test that goes by a string of letters or some other impenetrable name? Fine. But before you run off, get the facts. In addition to taking a more informed role in working with your doctor, you might save yourself some nasty surprises and needless worry. Before taking any test, always ask these questions:

- ☐ What does this test measure?
- ☐ Why do I need it?
- ☐ What could happen if I don't have the test?
- ☐ Are there any alternatives to the test?

- ☐ Will my health insurance pay the total cost for this test? If not, how much will it cost?
- ☐ How accurate is the test?
- ☐ How frequently does this test return false positives (the results show a problem that doesn't exist) and false negatives (the test says there's no problem, but there is)?
- ☐ How is the test performed?
- ☐ What kind of pain or "discomfort" is involved? Will four orderlies have to hold me down?
- ☐ What can go wrong?
- ☐ How should I prepare for the test?
- ☐ How will I feel after the test? (Can I return to work immediately? etc.)
- ☐ When will I get the results?
- ☐ Which lab is processing the test, and why did you choose that one? (Check to see if the lab is accredited by the Joint Commission at **www.jcaho.org** or by the College of American Pathologists at **www.cap.org.**)
- ☐ What's the ideal result that I want to get on this test?
- ☐ After taking the test and getting the results, what's the next step?

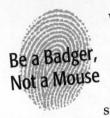

Be a Badger, Not a Mouse

When you're waiting for test results, don't assume that no news is good news. It's no news. Too many patients wait for the doctor to call them with results, or they figure that silence means everything's fine. Smart Patients always asks when the results will likely be in, and they call the office that day. And the next day, and so on, if the result isn't back yet. It's an extra reminder for us to call the lab if things are running behind. If the lab was supposed to send you a postcard with the result, it may have been lost. And in a bustling office, records can sit for a day or two without us knowing it. Be a nudge.

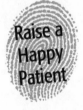

Raise a Happy Patient

We realize that this may be nearly impossible, but try to make your child's first doctor appointment a pleasant one, which does not involve a needle or a suppository or some equally less-than-fun event. Just as if her first dentist appointment involved a root canal, she might take a frowning view of future visits. Make a youngster's first association with doctors be a lollipop, not a rubella shot. Please emphasize that the visit isn't punishment for breaking the vase. Give her a special treat after the appointment. It'll prevent tears on everyone's part.

3

Let's Play Operation!

You're Having Surgery?
Use These Insider Tips to Sail Safely Through the OR

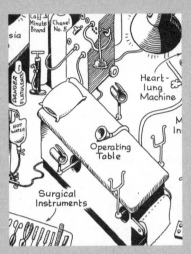

Have you had the pleasure yet?

We bet you have. Or maybe you're still looking forward to it.

We're talking about surgery, of course. We see it from the scalpel-wielding end just about five days a week, and it's still a thrill.

However, understandably, the patients on the other end of the adventure are a tad less enthusiastic. After all, they're asleep when all the interesting stuff happens. That's a bit ironic when you think about it, isn't it? They're undergoing one of the most important things that'll ever happen to them personally—one in which every little move can affect their lives—and during the whole thing they're sawing wood. Out like a light. Oblivious to everything and everyone. Could you imagine sleeping through your own wedding? Your child's graduation?

 Now, if you're on the table and have an anesthesia drip in your arm, you have a great excuse for snoozing. But a lot of patients doze through the whole process, starting six weeks before the surgery is even booked. They let their doctor make all the decisions, blindly assuming that everything will go smoothly because everyone will be looking out for them. They say, "Wake me when it's over," long before they step foot into the operating room, and they mean it.

Folks like this make us shiver in our scrubs. They don't realize that they're the surgeon's and anesthesiologist's biggest ally in making their surgery a success! That's because "having surgery" doesn't refer to the hour or so when you're in the operating room; it's a process that goes on for several weeks before and after the surgeon does his or her thing. And the main guard on duty during all that time is—drumroll, please—you.

Of any medical situation you'll ever face, having surgery is the only one where being a Smart Patient isn't just admirable, noble, and awe-inspiring, it's *absolutely mandatory*. When the inevitable happens, Smart Patients transform from savvy, educated consumers of health care into lean, mean,

Checklist: What Smart Patients Want to Know

When your doctor says, "You need surgery," that's your cue to put on your Sherlock Holmes hat and find out every pertinent detail—even the ones that seem too elementary to ask. Be inquisitive and be thorough, with a notebook, tape recorder, and your health care advocate right by your side (see the section "Advocating Advocates" on page 102 for details about this comrade-in-arms). Here are the key questions you should ask before undergoing any surgery—except maybe splinter removal.

- ☐ I know I've asked before, but can you review once again in lay terms why I need this surgery?
- ☐ What'll happen if I run for the hills and don't have it done?
- ☐ Can I peek at some of the data showing what happens if I "just say no"?
- ☐ What are the alternatives to surgery?
- ☐ What are risks of the surgery in the hands of a skilled practitioner? What if he or she is not skilled?
- ☐ Is there an alternative or newer way to perform the surgery that offers different pros and cons? If so, which method will you use and why? Any minimally invasive options? Are those better?

☐ Will the benefits be permanent? By the way, how long is "permanent"?

☐ Where is the absolute best place to have this surgery done besides here?

☐ How many of these specific surgeries does this hospital do a year?

☐ How long will I be in the hospital?

☐ Is it possible to do this on an outpatient basis, and if so, would that be smart?

☐ Can this be done under local anesthesia instead of general? (Don't get knocked out unless it's necessary, or the surgeon thinks it'll be most beneficial.)

☐ How many times have you performed this procedure? ("You're my very first!" is a bad answer.)

☐ How do your results in this operation compare with those of other surgeons?

☐ What kinds of complications do your patient's most frequently experience from this surgery? (Don't let the surgeon speak in generalities here.)

☐ What should I do and not do immediately before and after surgery? (Find out about food, alcohol, medications, sex, triathlons, and other activities.)

☐ Is the operation painful? How much pain will I be in after surgery? What painkillers will I be given during and after surgery? (Get drugs now; see the section "It's a Pain" on page 120.)

- [ ] How long will I be laid up after this surgery—meaning flat on my back or really unable to get around easily?
- [ ] How soon will I be able to drive? Do I need someone with me for the first twenty-four to forty-eight hours?
- [ ] What kind of scar (if any) will I have from the surgery? How long will it take to heal?
- [ ] How much time from work can I milk this for?
- [ ] Will I need physical therapy, and if so, for how long?
- [ ] What will my insurance cover? What will my insurance not cover? (Review your insurance plan ahead of time; it's a little easier to face surgery without worrying that you'll wake up $32,000 in debt.)
- [ ] What complications should I be on the lookout for after surgery, and what should I do if they occur?
- [ ] Who should I call after my surgery if I have questions, or if I experience something unexpected? (Get a specific phone number to call.)

fact-finding machines. They leave no proverbial stone un-
turned; they become detectives with the tenacity of Columbo
and Jessica Fletcher combined. (Hmmm, pairing a ratty trench
coat with pumps is an interesting look.)

Columbo

You'll probably feel most like Detective Columbo, come to think of it, since
you'll need to be sure to ask (and if necessary, rephrase and re-ask) questions
until you have all the information you
need. We'll impart their secrets—and
ours—in this chapter. Much of the territory we'll cover in the rest of this
book will be extremely useful when
you're having surgery, especially
the tips in chapter 6 ("Have a Happily Humdrum Hospital Stay") and chapter 7
("Why You Should *Always* Get a Second Opinion"). But the
tips in this chapter are the real must-dos whenever you have a
date with the surgeon.

Advocating Advocates

A Smart Patient isn't a lone force; he or she enlists a friend or
family member to act as a partner. Or, more specifically, as a
health care advocate. What is a health care advocate? Simply a
supportive, reliable person who serves as a second set of eyes
and ears in helping you get the best care. This person can accompany you to appointments, suggest questions to ask the

doctor, prevent oversights and mistakes, help you understand and remember care instructions, and also keep an eye on you to make sure you follow those care instructions between appointments.

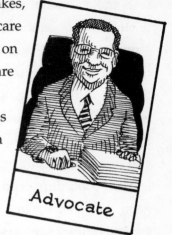

Advocate

Your advocate might take notes in the exam room, or she might sit in the waiting room and then discuss everything with you over coffee after the appointment—whatever works best. Surgery is certainly an apt reason to find a health care advocate, but it's an important move any time that you're being treated for a particular condition or disease.

A friend or relative with a medical background who's willing to help you could be a great choice, most obviously. But your advocate doesn't have to be an expert—just someone to stand by you and help you communicate with your doctor and whoever else is treating you. Your spouse can be a fine choice, of course, if he or she has the temperament for it. You want someone who's organized and will be a stress reliever. If the person you're sleeping with doesn't fit that job description, enlist another comrade.

Find the Best Surgeon

Minor surgery is an operation that someone else is having. If you're having any surgery, and especially if the best solution is a tricky operation, one that your doctor doesn't cautiously describe as "routine surgery," take the Smart Patient tip of finding the best doc for the job. Although gifted surgeons work in every hospital, you want the most specialized expert when you're having a potentially problematic procedure, and this surgeon may not be in your local area. Finding the best is worth the hunt, but it may take some detective work and research smarts.

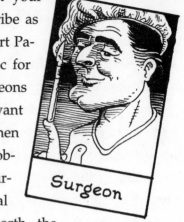

Surgeon

Right off the bat, recognize that you're going to judge a surgeon by a different measure than you used for your primary physician. For example, you're probably not going to have an ongoing relationship with this doctor, so you don't need to put much emphasis on his or her interpersonal cuddliness or bedside manner. Sure, you want to have some chemistry with the person who's going to be poking around your innards, but finding the charismatic doc with a flower in his lapel isn't your biggest concern. You're looking for sheer skill and experience. Think of the tech guy who fixes the computers in an office; you might not want to be stuck together for two hours in a Bennigan's booth, but he knows his bits and bytes.

So it's not a popularity contest. Then how do you choose the winner?

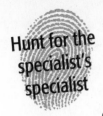

Hunt for the specialist's specialist You don't just want a doctor who is comfortable with performing a particular surgery as part of a wide repertoire, you want the surgeon who is obsessively focused on the specific technique that is the best choice for your specific surgery. Restated, you don't just want a gifted painter. You want the guy who paints only trees. *Sycamore trees.* In autumn. Every day, all day long. (See the sidebar "Are You the Guinea Pig?" on page 119.) For one example, cardiothoracic surgeons used to do all chest surgeries, from attaching new vessels to removing cancerous lungs. Today, one surgeon can gain so much experience with one specific heart valve's repair, that his or her patients have reproducibly fewer complications than the national average. For a second example, doctors who perform only nerve-sparing prostate surgeries have patients with lower rates of incontinence and sexual dysfunction. Aside from asking your regular doctor to point you to the maestro of this surgery, your own Internet research (see chapter 7 for info on this) can help you locate such a hyperspecialized surgeon. You just have to hope that one works at your hospital, or you might be in store for a road trip.

Use your doctor's referral as a starting point Your primary physician may recommend a surgeon that he or she has chosen many times for this surgery. There's a good chance your primary physician knows the doctor or that they're buddies. "She's excellent," your doctor might affirm, and in fact, this physician may be an excellent surgeon. But you can't just fly on that alone, especially if the surgery is highly complex. Your Smart Patient detective job is to find out if she's the most excellent surgeon you can choose for this particular operation. Ask your doctor for a few names, and give each of those surgeons a good looking over.

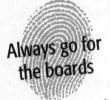

At a minimum, the surgeon must be board certified in the specialty involving your operation. It's a good sign if the surgeon is a fellow of the American College of Surgeons (ACS), indicated by the letters FACS after her name, which means she's been evaluated for ethical standards and professional competence. You can also visit **www.facs.org** (and click on "public information) or call 800-621-4111 and request a local list of ACS fellows.

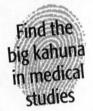

One insider way to find top specialists is to learn who is leading the medical research on the surgical technique for your specific health condition. Medline Plus can be a great Internet source for this. Further, by searching the more technical Medline database at **www.pubmed .gov,** you'll find studies from hundreds of medical journals. Searching for the specific name of the surgical technique is usually enough to cough up dozens. Be forewarned that these will be jargon-filled study summaries with 68-letter words and a lot of Latin, and, honestly, less interesting to read than car-ad disclaimers. But underneath the title of each study, you'll find the authors. Hopefully there will be one or two names repeated in several studies. Those doctors have a great shot of either being the practicing surgeons or clinical researchers who are more knowledgeable about your surgery than anyone else.

Armed with these names, take the studies to your doctor and ask if you'd be wise to consider having one of these specialists consult on your case. (We'll talk a little more about this in chapter 7, as it's useful for second opinions.) If your surgery is especially tricky or dangerous, and one of these specialists or hospitals has significantly greater experience in performing it than any surgeon you can find locally, you may consider traveling to have this doctor perform the surgery. Although some Smart Patients have enough savings to do this without hesitation, most don't have such deep pockets. Make no mistake, finding the absolute best surgeon (and leaving your insurance network to do so) can rack up bills that look like Bill Gates's bank statement. But whether you're rich or not so rich, always do this research so that you at least know your options. What's worth your money (or future debt), only you can say. In the long run, getting the best care is often less expensive than paying to correct the mistakes of less-than-perfect care. When it comes down to it, you might decide that having the absolute best brain surgeon is worth cashing in some of your retirement savings, since retirement might be a lot less fun after undergoing subpar brain surgery.

Scout for the cutting-edge procedure

Or, even better, the new one that doesn't involve any cutting. Do research and find out if there's a surgical technique for your specific problem that's more advanced, less invasive, or otherwise superior to the tried-and-true conventional procedure that your doctor may have suggested at the outset. If you can find a surgeon who's experienced in the latest technique, you may have safer surgery and heal faster.

For example, many surgeries that once required large incisions are now done laparoscopically, which uses tiny tubes to penetrate the skin. Similarly, there are new types of "keyhole" heart surgeries that require only a small incision, but not all heart surgeons are trained in using the new technique. (Tip: in hunting for the surgeon who's doing the newfangled procedure, well, let's just say that you're probably looking for a younger doc who's really good at video games.) That said, if you find a great surgeon who isn't using the newest technique, don't dismiss him or her. We see many patients who hear the words *minimally invasive* and then refuse to consider the conventional and proven surgery, even though the newer method may still have bugs. Get a second opinion to confirm whether the new surgery would really be best, and never push a surgeon to perform a minimally invasive technique if he or she doesn't really recommend it.

Surgical teams are well-oiled machines, and you want them performing with the finely tuned clockwork precision that they've perfected in hundreds of procedures. The last thing you want is to force them to practice a new method on you because you think it'll be safer.

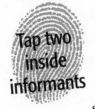

Tap two inside informants

If you're lucky enough to have a choice of surgeons at one or two area hospitals, go right to the source and get the scuttlebutt on them. Phone the department that'll handle your surgery, and ask a nurse for his or her opinion. (If you can do this face-to-face, such as when visiting a friend or relative, all the better.) The nurse will know the idiosyncrasies of the different surgeons, and, with some gentle and tactful Smart Patient questioning, she'll hint at which one she'd rather let take a scalpel to her.

Second, ask an anesthesiologist. If you phone the hospital's operating room between 3:00 P.M. and 5:00 P.M. on a weekday, there's a good chance that you'll find an anesthesiologist who's free. As you did with the nurse, say that you're about to undergo the specific surgery, and ask which surgeon he'd opt for if it was his abdomen going on the table. Anesthesiologists see every surgeon in action, and they know who's most careful.

Staff Nurse

SO, WHAT ARE YOU IN FOR?

If you have a surgery in your future, there's a good chance it'll be for one of these procedures. They're the most common procedures in the United States, according to the Agency for Healthcare Research and Quality (AHQR). In 2003, hospital patients underwent:

* 1.2 million cesarean sections
* 712,000 upper-GI (gastrointestinal) endoscopies (for diagnosing ulcers and other problems)
* 707,000 diagnostic heart catheterizations
* 676,000 angioplasties to widen heart arteries

Finding the Best Hospital

If you want a great meal, you go to a great restaurant, right? The same principle applies to safe surgery. (Except we mean you should go to a great hospital, not a great restaurant— although a hospital with a great cafeteria is certainly a perk.) While choosing a fantastic surgeon is critical, the caliber of the hospital or facility where you have the surgery is an equally important factor for success. That's because surgery exposes you to far more risks than the surgeon can control. Obviously, you should choose a Joint Commission–accredited hospital for your surgery. But here are some other tips for selecting a great hospital.

Check out a large teaching hospital

For any surgery that touches your organs or replaces any body part (that's our definition of a serious surgery), opt for a big hospital that, ideally, is affiliated with a university (of course we are biased because we practice in such facilities). The bigger the procedure, the bigger the hospital. Yes, size matters. Why? These hospitals have top-notch doctors and staffs on hand who are equipped to deal with complications. These backup players are critical, because often the primary operation isn't the problem at all, it's the complication that comes afterward that's the big, hairy, life-threatening deal. A small specialty hospital may be able to perform your heart surgery superbly, but make sure it has a team in place to give you kidney dialysis if something unforeseen happens. And does its OR bear any resemblance to the one on page 114? Surgery is all about the unforeseen possibilities, and Smart Patients take that into account when making choices about their surgeries. Everyone may not have immediate access to a large teaching hospital, so find the best one for you.

Don't forget small hospitals!

While large teaching hospitals may be getting a lot of the limelight here, don't forget small hospitals! We are fortunate in the United States to have many excellent small community and rural hospitals that provide outstanding care and service. To find the best hospital for you, check out the Joint Commission's Quality Check at **www**

.jcaho.org. Quality Check will help you search for the Joint Commission–accredited hospitals and other accredited health care organizations near you. In addition to an organization's accreditation status, Quality Check provides information about how well a hospital has complied with the Joint Commission's National Patient Safety Goals and other key clinical performance measures, such as heart attack care and pneumonia care.

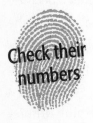

Check their numbers

Practice makes perfect, and perfect is what you want, right? The best two thumbs-up signs you can get for a surgery hospital are (1) it's accredited by the Joint Commission, and (2) proof that its doctors have done the specific surgery a gazillion times. Yes, you want a surgeon who's an old hand at that surgery (and an anesthesiologist who's worked with that surgeon many, many times), but you also want the hospital staff at large to be well versed in the procedure. Research has shown that, for several common operations, hospitals that perform at least a specific number of that operation every year have better success rates. To put it bluntly, patients who have these procedures done at high-volume hospitals are less likely to die or have unrecoverable complications. Your surgeon should be able to give you this info, as should the hospital's information line.

The following info comes courtesy of the Leapfrog Group **(www.leapfroggroup.org)**, which is one of the best things to happen to modern medicine since lollipops. It's a coalition of more than 170 large companies, most of them in the Fortune 500, who purchase health care for their employees in large scale. With their collective clout, Leapfrog makes things happen. For each operation named below, you'll increase your odds of returning home safely if you stick with a hospital that performs at least as many per year as the number given:

CAUTION • CAUTION • CAUTION •

OPERATION	MINIMUM NUMBER PER YEAR
Open heart surgery (of all varieties)	500
Heart transplant	9
Carotid-artery surgery	100
Esophagectomy	13
Mastectomy	25
Pancreatic cancer surgery	10
Pediatric heart surgery	100
Percutaneous coronary intervention	400
Prostate surgery	55
Repair/abdominal aortic aneurysm	30

Off-base Operating Room

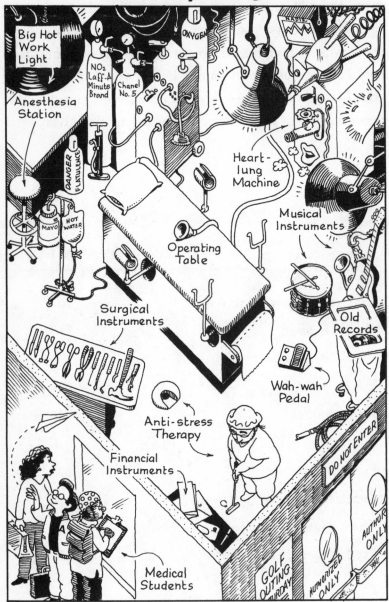

Go to your state database

Every state's Department of Health maintains a database that gives the success rate for certain procedures among hospitals and surgeons within its borders. Call your Department of Health or check its Web site's database for the procedure you're having. To find your state's general-information site, simply type the following in the URL-address box: www.[the two-letter abbreviation for the state name].gov. Some of these databases haven't been updated since the *Titanic* sank, so don't assume the information is flawless.

Have a Safe Snip

In chapter 5 we'll give you plenty of tips to make sure your hospital stay is serene and uneventful. Because surgery is one of the likeliest reasons you'll be in the hospital, make sure you get those insider tidbits before checking in. However, even in the hours before you're wheeled into the operating room, there are several key things you can do to boost your odds of leaving the hospital a happier and healthier person than the one who checked in. These things are second nature to surgical staffs, and they'll do everything they can to ensure that you come through surgery safe and sound. But to be a Smart Patient, always make triple sure that you:

Become comfortably numb— and no more

Don't worry too much about not waking up from the anesthesia. That risk is extremely small. In fact, for minimally invasive surgeries, you have about the same chance of dying from the anesthesia as you do from a haircut, which is about the same chance of dying from the embarrassment after a *bad* haircut. That said, general anesthesia (the kind that puts you to sleep, sometimes so deeply that a ventilator often controls your breathing) can cause nausea and has even been linked to lingering cognitive problems that have been detectable in some patients up to five years later. Therefore opt for the two least intrusive alternatives whenever you have the choice.

The first, and most mild, is local anesthesia, which is a shot that just numbs a body part. Above that, "twilight anesthesia"—or conscious sedation—produces a sleep that's not as deep as general anesthesia, but you'll remember nothing of the surgery afterward. And that's good, because the things we talk about . . .

Chat with the anesthesiologist before surgery

You need to meet the doctor face-to-face and give him or her some dirt on you, such as the last time you had general anesthesia, exactly how much you drink, what drugs you use and how often. People who "recreate" with substances can keep their habit hidden from lots of people, but they'd better be upfront with the anesthesiologist, because narcotics and other drugs can increase tolerance to se-

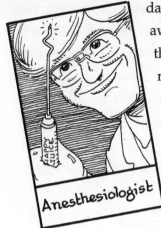

Anesthesiologist

dation, and they don't want to be wide awake when the surgeon asks for the knife. The anesthesiologist also needs to know how much you exercise, any allergies you have, and—for the umpteenth time during your hospital stay—every medication and herbal supplement you take.

What about those nightmarish stories you've heard about patients waking up during surgery? It's rare, but it happens. Talk to your anesthesiologist about this and decide if she should use a medical device that monitors your wakefulness.

Have the doc draw a picture

Surgery performed on the wrong limb? Or wrong person? Absurd. Unbelievable. Except in about 75 reported cases a year. Again, out of 25 million operations, 75 isn't a lot, but tell that to Joe, Larry, Michelle, Tina . . . The Joint Commission is on top of this problem and has developed a mandatory protocol for surgeons and organizations to follow for all surgeries. The surgeon must literally mark the site of your surgery (for example, left elbow, right side of abdomen, wherever appropriate) and should involve you, the patient, in the marking process. The surgical staff will double-check the site along with the surgeon immediately before the operation, and they'll review the X-rays again too. And the surgeon and surgical staff will also double-check your identity. Don't be worried if the surgeon asks you again right before surgery what your name is and what surgery you are there for. The surgeon hasn't suddenly contracted amnesia; he or she is just making sure that the right patient is getting the right surgery. And that keeps you safe.

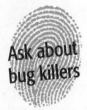

Ask about bug killers
Ask the surgeon if you should take antibiotics before the operation, as a precaution against infection. Patients don't need them before all operations, but it's important to ask.

Never shave your surgical site yourself
It's tempting, especially since you're probably bored, and it seems like common sense to give your doctors a clearer view of your skin. But shaving will leave you with thousands of tiny, invisible nicks that can increase your chance for infection, so let the team worry about defoliating you. For what you're paying for the surgery, believe us, it's included.

Enter the OR the way you entered the world
As in nekkid. And we don't just mean nude. We mean no makeup, no nail polish, no fake eyelashes, no rings, no bracelets, no lint in your belly button, no anything. Three fates can befall any detritus you have on your person during an operation: (1) they can get lost, (2) they can get in the way of the surgical team, and (3) they can get sewn inside

you. Actually, when one happens, all three tend to happen, so make sure you go in there sans extras. Besides, these extras can also harbor bacteria.

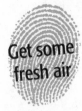

Get some fresh air

Ask for supplemental oxygen during and after the operation. A study found that receiving oxygen reduced infections in patients by 39 percent. Not bad for just inhaling.

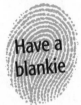

Have a blankie

Cold patients develop more complications, so make sure you request a blanket (if it won't get in the way) and ask your anesthesiologist to keep you warm during and after surgery, to ensure that you remain in a blissful state of normothermia. (Yes, *normothermia* is a real word; we recommend using it when complaining about the air-conditioning in a chilly restaurant.)

ARE YOU THE GUINEA PIG?

Pardon me, but you wouldn't mind too terribly if the twenty-nine-year-old resident performed his first operation ever on you, would you? You would? Well, how do you think we get new surgeons in this world? Somebody has to be the first patient. But we're with you all the way. We wouldn't let a newbie perform a serious procedure on us, either. Smart Patients know that it's a possibility, so they make sure it won't happen. But they're in the educated minority. A survey found that 60 percent of patients had no clue that they could be a resident's first dance partner in the OR. When asked, however, more than two-thirds didn't even want a new doc doing something as routine as inserting a tube in their throat.

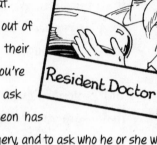

Resident Doctor

Spinal surgery? Only 1 out of 7 said they'd offer up their spines as testing ground. You're well within your rights to ask how many times the surgeon has performed the specific surgery, and to ask who he or she will delegate certain parts of the operation to. (You remember Hawkeye on M*A*S*H saying "Close for me" to the nurse, don't ya?)

One thing a Smart Patient doesn't do, however, is insist that a doctor do everything. It sounds prudent, but you don't want the department chair personally inserting your medication IV if she hasn't done it in twenty years. You can kindly ask the surgeon if he or she will actually be performing the surgery and request that residents or others only assist. You want them to follow their usual routine for your operation.

It's a Pain

Finally, to speed your recovery, don't leave the hospital or out-patient facility without a clear assurance that you'll be able to control any pain you might encounter. If that means taking home an enviable supply of the right pain medications, don't leave without them either. Ask your surgeon or doctor which variety of drugs will work best for you. And don't be afraid to take the painkillers if you need them; biting a stick went out with the Conestoga wagons. Here are the major choices:

Nonsteroidal anti-inflammatory drugs (called NSAIDs) NSAIDs, such as ibuprofen and aspirin, are used for mild to moderate pain. They also reduce swelling and soreness, but they can slow blood clotting and cause nausea, stomach bleeding, or kidney problems.

Opioids If you have severe pain after surgery, your doctor may prescribe an opioid such as oxycodone. These are strong drugs, and they can cause drowsiness, nausea, constipation, and problems with breathing or urinating. Codeine and morphine are two older drugs in this class that cause a lot of side effects. Some people are afraid of becoming addicted to opioids, but that risk is only about 1 in 7,000, and even then it's mostly a risk in patients who take them continually for chronic pain. So treat yourself right: use the strong stuff to get rid of the pain and get active.

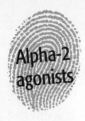

These drugs change your pain threshold. They're usually given only in intensive care units by IV, but newer versions are available by pill.

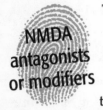

These work by the same mechanism as narcotics, but NMDAs are not addictive (although they are expensive and sometimes mood altering; ketamine and Dilaudid are two drugs in this class). They're commonly used in the recovery room and combined with a sedative, but they're also available in pills or liquids.

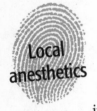

Local anesthetics are usually injected near your surgical incision to block the pain signals coming from that part of your body. They may also be given through an epidural, a small tube inserted in your back by an anesthesiologist. They can make you feel dizzy or weak but rarely cause other side effects.

By the way, you can now administer strong drugs to yourself when you're in the hospital with a new method called patient-controlled analgesia, or PCA. You control the amount of the drug that enters your body through an IV. Take comfort in knowing that you can be comfortable if you speak openly to your anesthesiologist about your needs and concerns before your operation.

Speaking of drugs, turn the page . . .

4
Prescription Drugs

Take Two and Pray You're Still Here in the Morning

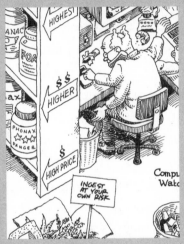

Smart Patients screen every single pill, lozenge, liquid, or needle before they put it into their bodies.

To be one of them, you need to become a very inquisitive detective every time a doctor hands you a prescription. You need to ask if you really need it, why you need it, when you need to take it, and how you need it—and, if it's an issue, where you need it. Being a Smart Patient also means knowing how to get medications on the cheap, without sacrificing quality or safety. In short, as a Smart Patient, you'll make medications work for *you*, while most other Americans have it the other way around.

We can hardly blame them, however, because putting our trust in prescription drugs is something most of us have learned to do all too easily. We live in a medication nation filled with hills of pills as the illustration of our neighborhood pharmacy (well, more or less) aptly shows. For almost every malady, real or imagined, there's probably at least one FDA-approved drug sitting in pharmacies and another barrelful in the pharmaceutical-industry pipeline on the way. Americans downed more pills and supplements every single day in 2005 than inhabitants of all developed countries gulped down in a month in 1950.

This evolution is a blessing in many ways, of course. For us as doctors, it's a fantastic feeling to be able give patients new medications that will improve their lives in some way, small or large. For some, it means having hope to fight an illness or syndrome for the first time. For others, it means a faster cure. For still others, it means an end to daily nausea or other side effects, while still controlling their condition. And let's not forget the thrill we get when we can tell a patient that the medication that cost $90 a month is now available for $20. Honestly, medications have given us some of our most satisfying moments as doctors.

You're waiting for the downside, aren't you? Well, millions of us, from Hollywood celebrities to stay-at-home parents, office execs to construction workers, share a tenuous

Phrantic Pharmacy

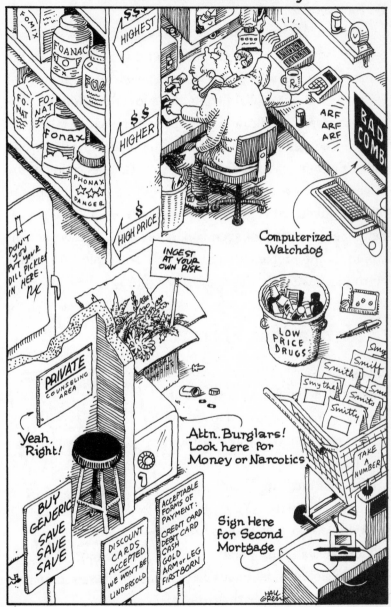

relationship with the prescription drugs we take every day. We have a tiger by the tail.

These drugs can do immense good. But if you or your doctor gets reckless or careless with them, these drugs can become more dangerous than a scorned lover. It's estimated that every year about 40,000 people die and 1.3 million are seriously hurt from medication mishaps, which include taking the wrong dose, getting the wrong prescription, mixing the wrong pills, or a combination of all three—sometimes even under the direction of a doctor. Only about half of all prescriptions are filled or taken correctly. Some physicians are fond of saying that for every dollar we spend on these drugs, it costs two dollars to fix the problem. Smart Patients don't join this merry-go-round. Take these tips to join their ranks.

Make a New Phriend

Your pharmacist is the least expensive and most accessible health resource you have. You can drop in to see him or her anytime you want, without an appointment. All consultations are free. In medicine, that's something extraordinary.

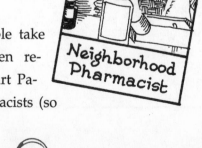

Neighborhood Pharmacist

Why do so few people take advantage of this golden resource? It baffles us. Smart Patients cuddle their pharmacists (so to speak) whenever possible; they know that building a relationship with this person is second in importance only to finding a great primary-care doctor. Your pharmacist has an amazing wealth of knowledge at her fingertips, which can mean at *your* fingertips. Many also have access to new technology that can answer questions (such as, is it safe to take this brand-new medication with this even newer medication?) in a blink. What's more, they get a soldier's-eye view of patients with similar conditions using different medications every single day (whether they like it or not). They see these patients improve. They see patients who complain about expected side effects, and they know which side effects could mean serious trouble, rather than just more time in the bathroom.

Pharmacists know many things that you don't. And, as difficult as it is for physicians to admit, they know many things that we don't. Most physicians take only one or two courses on pharmacology in medical school. The rest we learn from journals, from experience with patients, and from pharmaceutical salespeople who come a-knocking every single day of the week. (Sorry—please don't stop bringing us coffee mugs.)

Drug Salesperson

The point is, a good pharmacist can be more valuable than a great car mechanic. To put this power to work for you, follow these Smart Patient–tested tips.

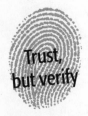

Think small, even at the biggest pharmacies

A Smart Patient knows the benefits of developing a personal relationship with a pharmacist. Your goal is to be on a first-name basis with your pharmacist, so that at some point two years from now, he'll mutter to himself, "Hmmmm... Jane's doctor has never prescribed this before, and it doesn't seem right, so I'd better shoot that doctor a call." Sure, it might seem easier to forge a personal relationship with one pharmacist at a smaller mom-and-pop pill dispensary rather than the new megadrugstore with thirty-nine aisles, but we've seen Smart Patients establish great relationships at the superstore pharmacies too. Even if the huge store has a rotating shift of six pharmacists, some of our patients know the one who is there every Wednesday by 9:00 A.M. after dropping off the kids but leaves by 3:15 P.M. to pick 'em up again.

The caveat here is to be certain that whatever pharmacy you choose, it should use the latest safety cross-checking software and medication-monitoring technology. Ask the pharmacist what he uses. After all, it's your health and safety.

Trust, but verify

Your pharmacist is a licensed professional, and that means you can check his or her credentials fairly easily. Each state has a board of pharmacy, which oversees and licenses guess who? And unlike teen drivers, pharmacists must have their licenses renewed every year or every other year. In appendix 3, Resources, there's a complete list of state pharmacy boards. If you call your state's office, you can confirm that your pharmacist is licensed in your state and also if he received disciplinary action for any reason.

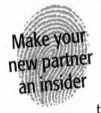

Make your new partner an insider
Slip your pharmacist one of the copies of the health journal you made way back in chapter 1. (See how handy that form is becoming?) Your pharmacy may or may not have the ability or inclination to include all of this info in your electronic record, but just having your pharmacist look it over while considering the medications you're getting is a great safety backup procedure.

Get your doctor to go digital
Some pharmacies allow doctors to write prescriptions electronically. Your doctor can punch in your prescription, and it'll be waiting for you when you arrive at the pharmacy. Best of all, this eliminates errors from misreading handwritten scripts (that's "doctorspeak" for prescriptions), and renewals are a snap. Ask your pharmacist if he has this capability, then ask your doctor to use it. In an emergency, having an electronic backup system with your prescription records could be a huge help. The 2005 hurricane devastation in New Orleans proved this point; people who used these systems had their lost drugs replaced and delivered to them much faster than other patients did.

DOES SIZE MATTER?

We have plenty of choices in pharmacies today. You probably can't drive two miles in your town without passing six drugstores and one new, colossal superpharmacy that could fit a small football stadium inside it. Big and small pharmacies come with their own pros and cons. Larger pharmacies are usually more automated, many are open 24-7, and they'll likely have every drug you could possibly need. Many are national chains with a central computer database, so they can fill your prescription at any location all over the country (a boon for frequent travelers). Smaller mom-and-pop pharmacies lack these amenities, but it can be easier to develop a personal relationship with the pill gurus there.

What about mail-order pharmacies? They're becoming far more common, and they offer two very enticing advantages: they're usually less expensive, and many will send you prescriptions or reminders at regularly scheduled intervals. Unless our health insurer required it, we wouldn't use a mail-order pharmacy that didn't allow us to communicate with a specific pharmacist there through its 800 number. Even then, as with car mechanics, you'd probably rather meet them in person than just trust them by the sound of their voices (our apologies to Click and Clack on radio's *Car Talk*).

Okay, so now you have a place to fill prescriptions. What Smart Patient detective work should you do when you're getting the prescription in the first place?

As you may have predicted, we have a checklist for you.

Checklist: The Pill Probe

Ask your doctor these questions every time she prescribes a new medication or increases the dosage of a drug you've been taking.

☐ What is this medicine for? This question might seem silly to you, but we see a staggering number of patients who have no idea why they're taking a certain medication. We also see plenty of new patients who have two or more health problems, and they're not sure which illness is being treated by which drug. Their doctor prescribed it, so they take it, end of story.

P. I. Kinsey Millhone

Being this uninformed invites trouble. Consider borrowing a tip from writer Sue Grafton's plucky private eye character, Kinsey Millhone, and give each drug its own index card.

☐ Does this medication replace anything else I'm taking?

☐ How do I take the medication? For example, should you take it with food or on an empty stomach? Does it need to be taken at certain times, such as every six, eight, or twelve hours? Do I need to wake up from sleep to take the pill? (This is rarely necessary, by the way.)

☐ How long do I take the medication? With some drugs, such as antibiotics, it's important to finish off the bottle even after you feel fine. With others, there is no set regimen; you can take as needed.

☐ What side effects can this drug cause, and how common are they? Which ones are the most dangerous?

☐ Is this drug new to the market? The federal Food and Drug Administration (FDA) can approve a drug for use after it's been tested successfully on a few thousand people for a relatively short period. When millions of people begin taking the drug, unforeseen problems can emerge, and this happens just often enough to warrant attention. If you're taking a relatively new drug, be even more attentive in telling your doctor about side effects.

☐ What are the odds that I'll have an allergic reaction to the drug? What are the likely symptoms and what should I do if that occurs? (Your pharmacist can access a frequency table for checking itching, vomiting, difficulty breathing, and so on.)

☐ How long have you been prescribing this drug for my condition? Are there any other medications for my condition that have been FDA approved more recently? If so, why is this drug the best choice?

☐ Is this medication safe to take with other medicines or dietary supplements I am taking? Now is the time to make sure that your doctor knows what you're currently taking, including all herbals and supplements.

☐ Can this medication cause any special problems in someone my age? This question is a prudent double check if you're older. A large study at Duke University found that more than 1 in 5 older patients were given prescriptions for drugs that could cause dangerous side effects in people older than sixty-five, while 1 in 25 were given three or more of these drugs at the same time. Americans older than age sixty-five buy 30 percent of all prescription medications and 40 percent of all over-the-counter drugs in this country, and they've also the most vulnerable to errors. The odds of having a dangerous drug interaction increase exponentially as you increase the number of drugs you take.

☐ Even if it's not highly dangerous, are there any other drugs, supplements, or foods I should avoid while taking this medication? What about alcohol? Do I need to wait several hours after taking the medication before drinking a glass of wine or beer, or do I need to cut out alcohol entirely?

☐ Any activities I should avoid (such as sitting in the sun) or should do (such as being near a bathroom)?

☐ Are you giving me a prescription for the brand name or the generic version of this drug? If the generic version is similar and costs less, could I take that?

☐ Does the prescription have all the refills, or will I have to contact you if I need to refill it?

Review the checklist with your pharmacist when you've actually getting the drug, both to prevent any errors and to get another expert's input. We just prescribe drugs; pharmacists dispense them every day, so they have insights that can be valuable to you. You'll also find forms for recording your prescription information in appendix 2. Make copies of these to take to every doctor's visit (along with all your pills), and ask your doctor to give you any details that you can't fill in yourself. You can then easily review specific questions in the checklist with your pharmacist; we guarantee that he or she will offer some new thoughts.

WHY THE BUZZ ABOUT GRAPEFRUIT JUICE?

Don't mix this drug with grapefruit juice! This strange warning has been circling in recent years. What could be so dangerous about the grapefruit, that tart bastion of citrus deliciousness? Well, it's a nerdy biochemical thing. To metabolize grapefruit, you use the same enzymes in your liver and lower intestines that you use to digest many drugs. If you eat grapefruit or drink grapefruit juice before or within eight hours of taking certain drugs—such as the cholesterol-reducing statin drugs (a common one being atorvastatin, or Lipitor)—those liver and intestinal enzymes will be occupied by the juice and not able to break down the drug. This means more of the drug will reach your bloodstream, which can increase its effect and chances of being toxic. Some patients try to harness this effect to save money; they'll split pills of a drug such as Lipitor and take it after drinking grapefruit juice to get the effect of a stronger dosage. This sounds pretty smart, but it's not Smart, if you know what we mean. For this to work, the pill must be made uniformly (many aren't), and your body needs to absorb the grapefruit juice and pill in perfect harmony, which is a mean feat. So don't try this at home, kids.

DANGER, WILL ROBINSON!

The next time you get medication from a pharmacy, your pharmacist might be a robot. More pharmacies are using "pick-and-place" robots to fill prescriptions and reduce errors. They fill prescriptions by reading bar codes, selecting the right pill or tablet from the right bin, and then bottling said pill or tablet in a container that's also bar-coded. (Bar codes are key in this process, we've noticed.) Pharmacists then check the prescriptions before they hand them out to patients. The automation saves time—a robot can prepare 1,500 prescriptions in an hour,

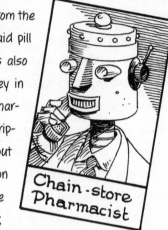

Chain-store Pharmacist

while it would take three panting pharmacists three hours to hit that tally. You probably won't see a mechanical arm whipping tirelessly in your corner drugstore anytime soon, but you never know.

A Milligram of Prevention...

There are a few other Smart Patient commandments concerning drugs. They not only make prescriptions much safer, they make them simpler to follow.

☛ Make sure your doctor and pharmacist know about every other drug, vitamin, nutritional supplement, and herbal remedy you're taking; as we'll discuss a little more saliently shortly, any of these could interact dangerously with medications.

☛ Get it in writing. Don't trust your memory. A 2005 study found that people's brains play an evil trick on them that can be dangerous when mixed with drugs. After being given a very clear order, such as "don't take this pill in the evening," they'll remember broad details—"pill," "evening"—but not the specific action that was requested. Guess what happens.

☛ Ask your doctor to write down the purpose of the medication on the prescription. That will help reduce the risk of a prescription mistake, as many drugs have similar names but much different uses (see the sidebar "Sounds Like Trouble" on page 155). As another safety measure, ask your doctor to write the drug's generic and brand names on the prescription.

☛ Fill the darn thing! About two in six prescriptions never get filled because people think they really don't need the medicine. A month later, we see them back in our office, sicker and contrite. We're not writing prescriptions to practice our penmanship, ya know.

☛ Keep your medications in their original bottles or packages to avoid getting confused. No offense to pills, but a lot of you look alike. It's also a good idea to keep a spare set of prescriptions with a week's worth of pills in a safe place, in case of emergencies.

☛ Don't take someone else's medication. We know, the stuff is expensive, and your friend has a coffee cup filled with the little black pills you need. Or think you need. Except those pills also look a lot like her birth-control pills. Don't try to save money this way. You're asking for more trouble than chasing a skunk.

☞ While you're at the pharmacy, read the label on your medication and make sure you have the right drug and the right dosage. If it's a familiar med, check to see that the pills look like the pills you've taken before. If anything seems iffy, holler.

☞ You know the instructions you get with your meds that's usually stapled to the bag? Many pharmacies now have a picture of the pill with the number or lettering of that particular medication. Open the container and make sure your pills match the information on the instructions.

☞ Ask the pharmacist if it is cheaper to use your prescription-drug health-insurance plan or pay cash. Some inexpensive medications can cost less than the co-pay. What a nice problem to have.

☞ Keep your medications separate from your pet's medications. Yes, we've seen it happen. And, yes, it is gross. Just when your heartworms thought they were safe.

☞ Toss all outdated medications, including nicotine or birth-control patches. We know this is a major bummer, but old pills can lose their effectiveness, making them worthless. They're also a dangerous source of mistakes, because the pills in that bottle may now be a motley mix of several drugs—as well as a few Tic Tacs and shirt-cuff buttons. Idle medication bottles in drawers tend to attract household flotsam over time. Don't crush or break any capsules or tablets unless your doctor or pharmacist tells you to. Some drugs may be absorbed too quickly if they're broken or if the capsule is removed before you swallow it.

☞ Use a memory jogger such as a timer or a pillbox. The more pills you're taking, the harder it is to remember when you took what or *if* you took what. Trust us on that. Keep a traveling stash, and pack more medicine than you'll need. We always get calls over the holidays and on summer vacations from patients who say, "I'm stuck here and completely out of my meds— please help!" Smart Patients wouldn't let this happen to them.

☞ Don't check your pills into your baggage at the airport. You'll go to Cleveland, they'll go to Tahiti. It's a hassle.

☞ Take your medication list with you when you go to the hospital, and make sure that the nurses and doctors have it (and know they have it!) before taking any new medications.

☞ Even if you're on a regular drug regimen, don't take any medication when you're in the hospital unless your doctor authorizes it.

☞ Have the doctor or staff nurse check your hospital ID bracelet before he or she gives you any medication, every time. Nurses hand out 600 pills a night. No offense to patients, but a lot of you look alike. More hospitals are using bar-code scanners on ID bracelets to double-check prescription orders. In fact, one of the Joint Commission's national patient safety goals requires health care workers to use at least two patient identifiers when administering your medications (neither can be your room number), to make certain that they are providing the right medication to the right patient.

☛ If you have to have a procedure or test that requires taking additional medicine or ingesting dye, remind your doctor, nurse, or technician of any allergies you have. Before you leave the hospital, review with the doctor, nurse, or pharmacist any drugs you're still taking. Update your Web-based medication list with any new prescriptions or changes in your drug plan. And don't forget to update **Your Health Journal** to include those new meds too.

☛ Don't poop out on us. About half of the patients who need drugs long term stop taking their medications within six months of their last doctor's visit. This is called "white-coat noncompliant"—patients take their meds only as long as the doctor's white coat remains vivid in their minds. It's sort of like driving fifty-three miles per hour for twenty minutes after the state trooper passes you on the highway.

☛ Don't store your drugs in the bathroom medicine cabinet. It can be a hot, moist place, like a subway in August. That can cause your pills to disintegrate or become pharmaceutically useless. Also, you know that every houseguest you have opens that mirror to see what you're hiding, don't you? During your next dinner party, leave a little note in there to greet them.

BID UNG AC. GOT IT?

When your doctor hands you a script, she knows you can't understand the little squiggles and abbreviations underneath the medication's name. Heck, most times you can't read the medication's name, never mind trying to translate those arcane, Latin-y abbreviations meant for the pharmacist's eyes. Doctors' bad handwriting isn't just the butt of jokes; there have been cases in which people actually died after their pharmacists misread the illegible scribbles and gave them the wrong drug or dosage. The Joint Commission has even issued an official "do not use" list of abbreviations that are common sources of errors.

Ask your doctor if he wouldn't mind spelling out the details instead of using that special shorthand, and to read the prescription out loud to you, so you'll have a fighting chance of translating it if necessary. If your doctor uses a computerized system to write prescriptions, still verify the name of the drug with her, as someone likely had to read the doctor's handwriting to enter it into the computer. Since you may still get scripts filled with hieroglyphics from time to time, use this cheat sheet to decipher them. Doctors typically write the name of the medicine first, then the form (say, capsule or tablet), dosage, amount (say, thirty tablets), directions for taking it, and finally the number of refills. Or, in medical shorthand:

* ac: before meals
* bid: twice a day
* dsp: amount to dispense
* hs: at bedtime
* prn: as needed
* qd: take daily

* sig: write on the label
* sos: may be repeated once
* stat: immediately
* tid: three times a day
* ung: ointment
* 2x: refill two times

Drugs? You Don't Know
What You're Mixing

There's one abbreviation that we're seeing way too much now: ADR. It means adverse drug reactions. These are complications patients face that are caused by mixing medications, or medications and supplements, or taking the drug in a way it wasn't supposed to be taken, or stopping a drug prematurely, or taking too large a dose, or mixing a drug with some odd genetic quirk that no one could have predicted you had. There are a ton of reasons. Adverse drug reactions are occurring more frequently for many reasons, and some are as obvious as an elephant on a freeway. There are more drugs available every day, pharmaceutical companies are selling more specific and more targeted drugs that still have unknown side effects, and patients are seeing more drug advertisements and asking their doctors if they should take them.

All of these factors encourage doctors to whip out their script pads ever more frequently. In fact, nearly two-thirds of all patient visits result in the doctor handing over a prescription, and more than half of all adults take two or more medications a day. In many cases, patients are too quick in asking for a drug, and sometimes

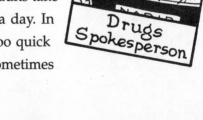

Drugs
Spokesperson

we're too quick in accommodating them. Safer non-drug treatments such as massage, hypnosis, or stress reduction could work just as well in many situations.

Drug alternatives are always worth investigating. The Smart Patient tips we've already given will do much to protect you, but we'd give this danger special attention, as it's afflicting more patients every year.

After you've asked your doctor the previous checklist questions, your pharmacist is your greatest ally in preventing adverse drug reactions. She'll use the pharmacy's computer system to check your new prescription against your drug history. The first danger sign the pharmacist is looking for is therapeutic duplication; that means taking two or more drugs that address the same problem but should not be taken together. For example, we often give patients two blood-pressure drugs, but it would be rare for us to intentionally mix two that are both water pills, since the compounded side effects could be dangerous.

The second thing the pharmacist's computer checks for is potentially dangerous interactions with all other drugs it has on file for you. This is the reason many men who somehow got a prescription for Viagra, even though they took certain heart drugs, got shot down at the pharmacy; the love drug could kill those men.

There's one danger that the computer often misses because it doesn't have enough specific info about you in the database: the foods you eat that could cause problems with the drug. We've already talked about grapefruit; for another example, some antibiotics become useless when mixed with milk.

In the following charts, you'll find the most common—and easily avoided—sources of adverse drug reactions. Keep this list handy, and review it whenever you bring home a new prescription—even after your doctor and pharmacist have vetted it with you.

ANTIBIOTICS

There are different classes of antibiotics, and your risk of a drug interaction often increases with the dosage of the drug you take. Antibiotics can be overused, so make sure that taking one is necessary to treat your condition.

DRUG	INTERACTS WITH	POSSIBLE EFFECTS
Tetracyclines	Minerals such as calcium, magnesium, and aluminum or dairy products	Binds antibiotics in your intestines, reducing their effectiveness
Tetracyclines	Anticoagulants	Decreases the effects of the anticlotting medication

DRUG	INTERACTS WITH	POSSIBLE EFFECTS
Erythromycin	Theophylline, an asthma drug	Increases levels of the asthma drug
Erythromycin	Statin drugs such as Lovastatin, and many other cholesterol-altering drugs	Increases risk of muscle aches and soreness
Erythromycin	Anticonvulsant drugs such as carbamazepine	Increases the effect of the anticonvulsant medication
Erythromycin or azithromycin	Antiarrhythmic drugs such as sotalol or dofetilide	Causes dangerous heart rhythms
Fluoroquinolones (such as Cipro)	Mineral supplements such as calcium, magnesium, and aluminum	Reduces effectiveness of antibiotics

CAUTION · CAUTION · CAUTION ·

ANTIDEPRESSANTS

Commonly used antidepressants include the monoamine oxidase (MAO) inhibitors Nardil (phenelzine) and Parnate (tranylcypromine), and selective serotonin-reuptake inhibitors (SSRIs) such as Prozac (fluoxetine). As mentioned below, these drugs should not be taken together.

DRUG	INTERACTS WITH	POSSIBLE EFFECTS
Selective serotonin-reuptake inhibitors	St. John's wort	Increases effects of SSRIs, which could result in too much serotonin being produced, causing jitters and other side effects
Selective serotonin-reuptake inhibitors	MAO inhibitors	Increases effects of SSRI drugs, which could be fatal
MAO inhibitors	Decongestants such as pseudoephedrine, or diet pills with ma huang and many other diet aides	Can increase blood pressure dangerously, risking a heart attack or an aneurysm

DRUG	INTERACTS WITH	POSSIBLE EFFECTS
MAO inhibitors	Certain cheeses, herring, and beverages such as Chianti wine	Dramatically increases blood pressure
MAO inhibitors	Demerol (meperidine) and other prescription pain relievers that have a narcotic component like Percocet and Tylenol #3	Can cause serious cardiovascular and blood-pressure instability and/or coma

CAUTION • CAUTION • CAUTION •

BLOOD-PRESSURE MEDICATIONS

Blood-pressure medicines can help you keep your blood pressure at healthy levels, but they can interact with other medications as well as with grapefruit juice and potassium.

DRUG	INTERACTS WITH	POSSIBLE EFFECTS
Angiotensin-converting enzyme (ACE) inhibitors such as lisinopril	Specific classes of diuretics such as spironolactone— so-called potassium-sparing diuretics	May increase potassium levels dramatically, which can cause irregular heartbeats or death
ACE inhibitors	Potassium	May increase levels of potassium
Some calcium-channel blockers	Grapefruit juice	Increases absorption of the calcium-channel drug, and thus increases the effect, leading to rapid drop in blood pressure

CAUTION · CAUTION · CAUTION ·

BLOOD THINNERS

Blood thinners such as warfarin have a higher risk of interactions than many other drugs.

DRUG	INTERACTS WITH	POSSIBLE EFFECTS
Warfarin	Antibiotics such as clarithromycin or erythromycin	Can increase the effect of warfarin to cause abnormal bleeding
Warfarin	Herbs, especially those starting with a *g*, such as ginseng, glucosamine, ginkgo biloba, garlic, and ginger	Can increase the effect of warfarin to cause bleeding
Warfarin	Spinach and other leafy greens	The large quantities of vitamin K in these foods may decrease the effects of warfarin, which could allow blood clots

DRUG	INTERACTS WITH	POSSIBLE EFFECTS
Warfarin	Miconazole (found in over-the-counter yeast-infection treatments)	Increases risk of bleeding and bruising

CAUTION · CAUTION · CAUTION ·

COLD AND SINUS MEDICATIONS

It's easy to assume that over-the-counter medications are always safe, but remember that they can interact with other medicines. Remember to tell your doctor or pharmacist about the OTC medicines you're taking before you begin taking a new prescription drug.

DRUG	INTERACTS WITH	POSSIBLE EFFECTS
Nyquil or other alcohol-containing cold medications	Antihistamines or alcohol	Strong sedative effect that could cause a coma, or worse
Antihistamines	Kava or other antianxiety meds	Sleepiness, pronounced sedative effect
Antihistamines	Some sleep aids such as Sominex	Pronounced sedative effect

PAIN RELIEVERS

Pain relievers, while commonly taken, can also interact with other medications.

DRUG	INTERACTS WITH	POSSIBLE EFFECTS
Acetaminophen	Alcohol	Can cause liver damage if used chronically
Aspirin	Alcohol at same time (not next morning)	Increases risk of upset stomach, irritation, and heartburn
Aspirin	Celebrex or other nonsteroidal anti-inflammatory drugs (NSAIDs), such as ibuprofen	Increases risk of gastric bleeding, and also reduces protective effects of aspirin against heart attack and stroke
Aspirin	Insulin	In high doses, can affect blood-sugar levels

DRUG	INTERACTS WITH	POSSIBLE EFFECTS
Celebrex	Nonsteroidal pain relievers and prescription anti-inflammatory drugs such as ketoprofen and diclofenac	Increases risk of gastrointestinal bleeding
Ibuprofen or indomethacin	Anticoagulants such as warfarin	Can cause irritation of the gastrointestinal tract or gastric bleeding
Ibuprofen or indomethacin	Some high-blood-pressure medications	May reduce effects of blood-pressure medications

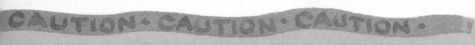

ORAL CONTRACEPTIVES

Although there are dozens of oral contraceptives available, be aware that taking other drugs can decrease their effectiveness.

DRUG	INTERACTS WITH	POSSIBLE EFFECTS
Oral contraceptives	Antibiotics such as penicillin and tetracycline	May reduce the effectiveness of oral contraceptives

DRUG	INTERACTS WITH	POSSIBLE EFFECTS
Oral contraceptives	St. John's wort	May reduce the effectiveness of oral contraceptives
Oral contraceptives	Ginseng	May increase the potency of estrogen in oral contraceptives, causing estrogen-related side effects such as weight gain or breast cancer (if long-term use)

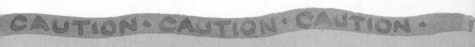

CAUTION • CAUTION • CAUTION •

OTHER MEDICATIONS

DRUG	INTERACTS WITH	POSSIBLE EFFECTS
Accutane, an acne medication	Vitamin A	Can result in hair loss, dry scaly skin, and other side effects
Antianxiety drugs such as Xanax and Valium	Alcohol	Excessive sedation

DRUG	INTERACTS WITH	POSSIBLE EFFECTS
Flagyl, an antifungal drug	Alcohol	Flushing reaction where you feel hot and flushed, and heart rate increases
Fosamax (and lots of other drugs, too)	Food	Reduces the absorption of the drug, thereby reducing effectiveness. Ask your pharmacist!
Nitroglycerin	Alcohol	Can cause cardiovascular collapse and severe hypotension, or low blood pressure
Sinemet, used for Parkinson's disease	Vitamin B_6	Decreases the effectiveness of the medication
Statins such as Lipitor, Pravachol, Zocor, Crestor, etc.	High doses of vitamin C and/or E (more than 200 mg of C or 100 IUs of E)	Inhibits anti-inflammatory effect of statin drug
Viagra	Nitroglycerin	Can cause significant drop in blood pressure, which can be fatal

SOUNDS LIKE TROUBLE

Hundreds of drugs have scarily similar names, and, more scarily, they occasionally get mistaken for one another. Here's a sampling of a few that could easily be crisscrossed by an imperfect humanoid. The Joint Commission is focusing on this problem too; they require health care organizations to identify and review (at least once a year) a list of lookalike/soundalike drugs and take action to prevent mix-ups.

Is this a prescription for...	Which is a drug designed to treat...	Or are you supposed to take...	Which is a drug that treats...
Lamisil (terbinafine)	Nail infections	Lamictal (lamotrigine)	Epilepsy
Zyrtec (cetirizine)	Allergies	Zyprexa (olanzapine)	Mental conditions
Serzone (nefazodone)	Depression	Seroquel (quetiapine)	Schizophrenia
Celebrex (celecoxib)	Arthritis	Celexa (citalopram)	Depression
Ritalin (methyl-phenidate)	Attention-deficit disorders	Methadone (dolaphine)	Narcotic withdrawal and dependence
Taxol (paclitaxel)	Ovarian, breast, and non-small-cell lung cancer	Taxotere (docetaxel)	Breast cancer, prostate cancer, non-small-cell lung cancer, and other types of cancer

Is this a prescription for...	Which is a drug designed to treat...	Or are you supposed to take...	Which is a drug that treats...
Velban (vinblastine)	Lymphomas, numerous cancers, histiocytosis, idiopathic thrombocytopenia purpura (ITP)	Oncovin (vincristine)	Leukemia, lymphoma, breast and lung cancers
Xanax (alprazolam)	Anxiety	Zantac (cimetidine)	Stomach ulcers
Prilosec (omeprazole)	Heartburn	Prozac (fluoxetine HCL)	Anti-depressant
Advair (fluticasone propionate and salmeterol)	Asthma	Advicor (niacin extended-release and lovastatin)	Abnormal cholesterol levels
Diflucan (fluconazole)	Yeast infections	Diprivan (propofol)	Sedative
Heparin	Blood clots	Hespan (hetastarch in sodium chloride)	Shock, following serious injury, bleeding, or burns

The 411 on OTCs

As shown in the adverse drug reaction charts on the previous pages, nonprescription drugs—even old stalwarts such as aspirin—can still put a hurting on you if abused or taken with the wrong counterpart. The thousands of over-the-counter drugs in your local pharmacy deserve the same cautious respect that prescription medicines deserve, even if they are right next to the Band-Aids. The next time you need an OTC drug, head back to the pharmacy instead of just running in the drugstore and making a quick grab. Your good buddy Mr. or Ms. Pharmacist can be especially helpful in helping you make a wise purchase—and, as always—a safer one. Remember, they see hundreds of people file in and out with all sorts of ailments. Given this daily focus group, they likely have an inkling of the over-the-counter drug that works best for a particular problem. But don't just hold up the elixir and ask, "Is this one good?" Tell your pharmacist the full story:

☛ Who the medicine is for. Is it for you, your five-year-old child, or your seventy-three-year-old parent? No fair sharing unless you tell the pharmacist.

☛ What symptoms you're trying to treat, how severe they are, and how long they've existed.

☛ What health conditions you or the would-be medicine taker have.

☛ What makes the symptoms better or worse.

☞ What else you've already taken or tried to cure the problem, and if it helped.

☞ What other drugs that medicine, supplement, vitamin, or ointment will meet in your or the intended's bloodstream.

In tapping your pharmacist this way, you'll greatly reduce the odds that you'll be in the ER later that evening with stomach bleeding, or the chance that you'll be up at 3:00 A.M. telling your equally miserable spouse, "I spent fifteen bucks on this junk, and it has not helped at all."

Too Much of a Good Thing

It's no secret that doctors prescribe antibiotics far too frequently in the United States, and that patients often ask for them—adamantly—when they're most likely unnecessary. Have you ever tried to send patients home with a miserable cold with nothing other than a prescription to drink fluids and watch TV for a few days? It makes folks mad. They want the good stuff, the little orange germ killers. Many have heard the fact that antibiotics kill only bacteria, not viruses (although some get this backward), so those pills can do absolutely nothing to kill the rhinovirus that's wreaking havoc in their nose.

Some have even heard another fact: Every time you take an antibiotic, you increase the chance of developing stronger, drug-resistant bacteria. That hurts all of us. And it's a reason why our most powerful antibiotics are not helping some patients. That scares the stuffing out of many health care professionals. And it scares Smart Patients.

Don't ask for antibiotics unless you and your doctor both agree that they're absolutely necessary. Likewise, always question an antibiotic prescription, and ask if there's an alternative to murdering millions of innocent bacteria in your intestines. When you take them, finish the bottle, even if you have to keep taking them for two weeks after you're well. You need to annihilate all of the bacteria, including the hardiest strains, because the surviving bugs will learn how to beat the antibiotic in much the same way that you learn how to avoid a speed trap. Yes, bacteria are smart. And the last thing we need are stronger, smarter bacteria in the world.

One more scary but also kind of fascinating reason you should avoid taking unnecessary antibiotics: Your intestine is home to many kinds of bacteria; there are more than 500 varieties that could kill you, and would if they got a fair chance (the little monsters). Luckily, your intestine is full of good bacteria, too, and they stop the villains from running amuck. If you take an antibiotic you don't need, you might wipe out the bacteria that wear the white hats and leave the black-hatted bugs to take over Dodge City. Mayhem could ensue. So trust your doctor when she tells you that you don't need an antibiotic. Your friendly intestinal bacteria will thank you.

How Much? Per *Pill*?

If Donald Trump wants to become a pauper in six months, all he needs to do is lose his prescription-drug insurance and then get a chronic illness.

True story: A guy was ahead of us in a pharmacy line, and his insurance company was refusing to cover his prescription, saying that his doctor had exceeded the recommended dose. He needed it, he pleaded with the pharmacist—one he did not know by name. The man said he'd begin suffering withdrawal if he stayed off the medication for another day.

"Well, you could just pay the full price for two weeks' worth, then try to get it back from your insurance company," the pharmacist said.

"How much is it?" the man asked.

The pharmacist looked in a binder and then tapped on a calculator.

"It's $288."

"For . . . two . . . weeks?" the man said.

"Well, fifteen pills, so two weeks and a day," the pharmacist responded. "I'll stay sick," the guy said angrily and stalked out.

We felt for him.

Smart Patients don't get into this mess. They know the best ways to cut the high costs of drugs:

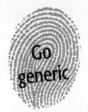

When a drug's patent life is over (commonly twenty years after discovery, and six to eight years after it has been on the market), other companies can sell the drug, and this usually cuts the drug's price to just a bit over what it costs to manufacture it. So get the cheaper generic version whenever one is available.

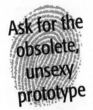

If there is no generic equivalent, ask your doctor if there's another form or an older form of the drug that's cheaper. Pharmaceutical companies continually refine drugs to keep customers like you happy, and often that means creating longer-lasting drugs that need only one dose instead of two or three taken throughout the day. When patients switch to the new one-dose version of a drug, its multi-dose forebearer becomes yesterday's news—and often drops in price.

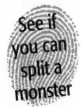

Pharmaceutical companies often charge the same amount per pill regardless of its potency; that means you'll pay two bucks for a pill whether it's 10 mg or 40 mg. If the drug is made uniformly (and many are not, so check with your doctor and your pharmacist), you might save money by getting the most powerful dosage available and splitting the pills into halves or quarters. (And inexpensive pill splitters are available that make this task easy.)

Bargain with your buddy

Pharmacies are businesses, and few people realize that prices are negotiable. If you tell your pharmacist that you saw the drug you need for less money at a competing pharmacy—and you can prove it with an advertisement or digital photo, if he's not quite the bosom buddy you're shooting for yet—the pharmacist might match the price.

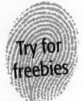

Try for freebies

Ask your doctor for drug samples. Drug reps hand them out, and most physicians save them for patients who are truly needy. If that's you, ask for the free samples, but be certain that you get clear, written instructions from your doctor on how to take the

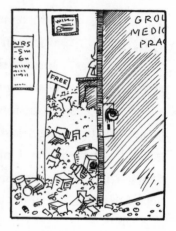

drug. You won't have a bottle label to read.

Use the forklift

If you'll need a particular medication on an ongoing basis, and it has a long shelf life, buy the pills in bulk.

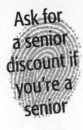

Ask for a senior discount if you're a senior

(Or close enough to pass for one.) Hey, you earned it. Be too proud on matters that won't save you cash.

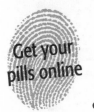

Get your pills online

If you find a reputable Internet pharmacy that will ship you quality-tested authentic medications, give it a good looking over. Some online pharmacies have lower prices than even the cheapest mail-order outfits. But remember, you want to do business only with an online pharmacy that has a real live person you can speak with on the phone whenever you want. And you only want one that's been certified by the Verified Internet Pharmacy Practice Sites (VIPPS). This means it has met standards set by the National Association of Boards of Pharmacy. If you don't see a VIPPS seal of approval, check the National Association of Boards of Pharmacy site at **www.nabp.net/vipps/intro.asp** to see if the pharmacy is licensed and in good standing. Avoid sites that fail both tests, that may get their drugs from places outside the United States (where testing standards may be poor), or that don't require a prescription for prescription drugs.

Remember that much of the world's pharmaceutical supply is counterfeit. If you suspect that a site is illegal or sketchy, report it to the FDA at **www.fda.gov/oc/buyonline/buyon lineform.htm.**

Tap the plastic

A lot of pharmaceutical industry execs aren't the fat cats some imagine them to be (see right); many have created drug discount cards that will save you up to 40 percent on medications. These cards are issued by specific pharmaceutical companies such as Pfizer, Eli Lilly, AstraZeneca, Johnson & Johnson, and Janssen to offer

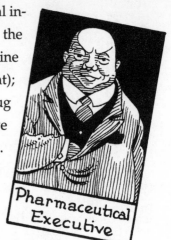

Pharmaceutical Executive

financial assistance to people who have difficulty paying for their drugs. These programs are generally available to needy people with low incomes. Following is a sample of drug discount-card programs:

Medicare-Approved Drug Discount Cards People with Medicare but without private prescription-drug coverage who earn less than $12,570 per year (or $16,863 for a married couple) can use this discount program for an annual cost of $30. Info: **www.medicare.gov,** 800-MEDICARE.

Together Rx Access This program offers discounts for more than 275 drugs to people with low incomes who don't receive Medicare or have other drug insurance. Info: **www.trxaccess .com,** 800-444-4106.

Johnson & Johnson Partnership for Prescription Assistance (PPA) J&J has one of the largest discount drug plans. Info: **www.pparx.org**, 888-4PPA-NOW.

Pfizer Pfriends Program Pfizer offers savings of up to 50 percent on its drugs. Info: **www.pfizerhelpfulanswers.com**, 866-776-3700.

U Share Prescription Drug Discount Card U Share is sponsored by the United HealthCare Insurance Company along with a few drug companies. Info: **www.usharerx.com**, 800-707-3917.

AstraZeneca Foundation Patient-Assistance Program AstraZeneca's program taps you into more than 275 public and private drug-discount programs. Info: **www.astrazeneca-us.com**, 800-424-3727.

LillyAnswers This program can save you up to $600 a year on Eli Lilly medications. Info: **www.lillyanswers.com/en/index.html**, 877-RX-LILLY.

Janssen Patient Assistance Program The pharmaceutical company provides free Janssen drugs to low-income Americans. Info: **www.janssen.com**, 800-652-6227.

Don't let the insurance company push you around

Flip to chapter 10 for more tips on this.

ONLINE RESOURCES

Visit the following Web sites to learn more about the medicines you're taking, including how to avoid adverse drug reactions.

Ask NOAH: Pharmacy/Drugs and Medications
www.noah-health.org/en/pharmacy/index.html
This site, developed by four New York library associations to provide accessible health information to the public, includes links to dozens of pharmacy- and medication-related Web pages.

Center for Drug Evaluation and Research (CDER)
www.fda.gov/cder/drug
This site, part of the FDA's Center for Drug Evaluation and Research, includes information about prescription and over-the-counter drugs, drug safety, and links to major drug-information pages.

Division of Over-the-Counter Drug Products
www.fda.gov/cder/Offices/OTC/default.htm
This site, part of the FDA's Center for Drug Evaluation and Research, has information about over-the-counter drugs and their safe use.

Drugs.com
www.drugs.com
This site includes a database with drug information drawn from three leading medical-information suppliers; provides a free drug-information service for both prescription and OTC drugs.

FDA Kids' Page
www.fda.gov/oc/opacom/kids
This site, sponsored by the U.S. FDA, is designed to help children learn more about drug and food safety.

SafeMedication
www.safemedication.com
This site, sponsored by the American Society of Health System Pharmacists, includes information for consumers about using medication safely and appropriately.

United States Pharmacopeia (USP)
www.usp.org
This site, part of the United States Pharmacopeia, provides information about safely using drugs to treat children.

Institute for Safe Medication Practices
www.ismp.org/Pages/Consumer.html
Offers info to reduce the risk of medication errors.

Medline Plus
www.medlineplus.gov
We gave you this one before, but it's a good resource for prescription and over-the-counter drugs.

5

How to Case a Hospital

Use an Expert's Eye to Find the
Best Hospital for Your Specific Goals—
and Learn Why One Size Does Not Fit All

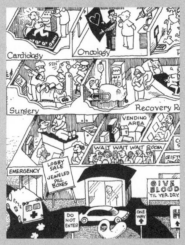

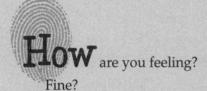**How** are you feeling?

Fine?

Never better?

You need to find a hospital. The perfect time to scout for the best hospital is when you don't need one. And doing it now will let you be objective and unhurried in evaluating which area hospital would be your go-to choice. The absolute worst time to make this decision is exactly when most people do; they don't give it a thought until a paramedic is looking them in the eye and asking, "Do you have a preference of which hospital you want to go to?"

"Huh?"

Wham! From the very first moment of a health crisis, you're unprepared and not in control.

Sure, we already talked about evaluating your primary-care doctor by the hospitals where he or she enjoys coffee. And in discussing surgery in chapter 2, we talked about needing to find a qualified Joint Commission–accredited hospital that's highly experienced in doing the procedure you need to have done. But what about when you or a family member needs emergency care? Or you need to recuperate from a procedure? Or you need to have a battery of tests done? This decision gets hairier than a barbershop floor because the hospital where your doctor is the kingpin may be excellent at total hip replacement, but it might be the absolute last place you'd want to go if your heart was calling it quits at 1:00 A.M. Likewise, the hospital that was unbeatable when you were in an auto accident and needed emergency care to stop bleeding might not be the best joint to be admitted for cancer care.

You should consider these factors at least as well as you consider which automotive shop to take ol' Bessie for her 30,000-mile checkup. Don't leave your hospital choice to chance.

Smart Patients, as you can imagine, never do.

• • •

A ctually, if you're like 95 percent of the U.S. population, you have several choices of hospitals beyond the two or three that are closest to you. Smart Patients choose by always keeping two criteria in mind: (1) Which hospital is best qualified to save my life in an emergency? and (2) Which hospital is best qualified to treat me for non-emergencies or for the things I am likely to need? These might turn out to be the same place. But sometimes they don't.

It's easy to forget that hospitals are businesses. As with all businesses, some are run better than others. Some have better staff morale, higher day-to-day standards, and cleaner bathrooms. Better or healthier cafeterias and nicer elevator music. Some are saddled with politics and clique wars. Some provide reasonable service and safety, while others offer patient safety and service worthy of a five-star hotel. And a few may even look like the hospital on the next page. We'll tell you how to get the best. And we'll also tell you the specific questions you'll need to ask as you investigate and query the hospital personnel. To win these folks over, you may want to take the soft approach and be a gentle inquisitor; think of Charlie Chan gently coaxing information out of his subject.

The Hospital from Heck

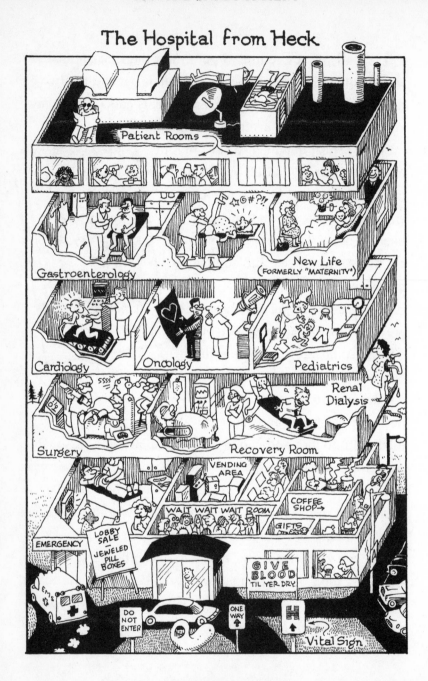

Every workplace deals with some of these factors, to be sure. But there's a key difference. In most jobs, such human peccadilloes usually don't mean the difference between your life and death, or at least not directly and immediately. Unless your work involves making nuclear warheads, all-season tires, or lightly cooked pork products, your team can probably churn out some pretty careless and slapdash work before it endangers people's lives. Hospitals don't have that leeway.

How should you screen your area hospitals to make sure you tap the best one in your predicted circumstance? Fortunately, hospital excellence is the very thing that the Joint Commission specializes in. And in our careers as doctors, well, we've seen just about everything, so we'll tell you exactly what you need to know. By applying the following Smart Patient test to each hospital, you'll find the best place for you and your family.

What about word-of-mouth referrals from friends, relatives, and any person you might know who works in health care? They are certainly valuable. But not nearly as valuable as the facts you'll get by asking your hospital candidates the following questions.

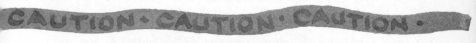

THE SMART PATIENT HOSPITAL TEST

You'll know the answers to some of the following questions off the top of your head, others you'll find on the hospital's Web site, and a call to the hospital's main number will fill in any stragglers. The questions are ordered from most important to least, so if you circle no in response to the first three or more, move on. That hospital isn't worth your time or your money. If you answer yes to eight or more, including the first three questions, you might have a love connection.

Y / N   Does your primary-care doctor treat patients at this hospital?

Y / N   Will your health insurance cover treatment at this hospital?

Y / N   Is the hospital accredited by the Joint Commission? And is its accreditation current and in good standing? You can check a hospital's status on www.qualitycheck.org or by calling 630-792-5000. If a hospital is unaccredited, it may mean it has failed to meet minimum standards in preventing medical mistakes, managing meds correctly, preventing infection, or other major safety areas. It may also mean the hospital has dropped its accreditation.

Y / N   Is it a "magnet" hospital? Facilities with a high number of well-trained nurses earn this status from the American Nurses Credentialing Center. Click on www.nursingworld.org/ancc to see if the hospital made the cut.

Y / N   Does the hospital employ full-time intensivists (doctors who specialize in treating critically ill patients) and full-time hospitalists (doctors who treat only hospital patients, and have no private practice)?

Y / N   Is it a teaching hospital affiliated with a major medical university? As we've mentioned, these hospitals tend (*Tend!* Please, no hate mail!) to have the most experienced staffs and the most thorough resources. See "Teaching Hospitals: What's the Big Deal?" opposite.

Y / N   If residents participate in patient care, are they adequately supervised by the attending physicians? In most teaching hospitals, most patients are treated by residents. However, that doesn't mean the residents are the sole providers of care or that the residents are directing the care unsupervised.

Y / N   Does the hospital specialize in your specific condition? If you need treatment for a particular disease or disorder, a small specialty hospital may offer you better care than a large general hospital, but not if you have another preexisting complication or serious condition, or suffer a complication.

Y / N   Does the staff use a computerized system to enter patient orders and prescriptions? Properly using this technology is far safer than writing everything. It can prevent as many as two-thirds of medication errors alone.

Y / N   Has your primary-care doctor or his or her family member ever been treated at this hospital for a serious problem as an inpatient? You can ask the doctor directly, or coax this detail out of his or her staff. You *are* making friends at the doctor's office, right?

Y / N   Does the hospital look generally clean and well kept? Trust your instincts.

Teaching Hospitals: What's the Big Deal?

You've heard it plenty of times, and more than once from us, we know. Teaching hospitals may offer better care and more cutting-edge treatment than the hospitals that see nary a med student. They have a responsibility to incorporate the latest techniques and medical advances into their treatments because they're training tomorrow's doctors. That translates into an advantage for you if you're undergoing a tricky surgery or otherwise present a challenging case to your doctor. Having student doctors around also keeps doctors on their toes, since the young upstarts are always asking challenging questions ("Why did you just order that test?").

FIND CARE THAT'S A WORLD APART

The Joint Commission accredits health care organizations internationally too. So if you're traveling abroad, know before you go. Check out the accredited hospitals in a foreign country by going to the Joint Commission Resources Web site at **www.jointcommission international.com** and clicking on "JCI-Accredited Organizations." There are Joint Commission International–accredited hospitals in Austria, Brazil, China, Czech Republic, Denmark, Egypt, Germany, India, Ireland, Italy, Mars (just seeing if you were still reading), the Philippines, Saudi Arabia, Singapore, Spain, Thailand, Turkey, and the United Arab Emirates. And the number of countries with JCI-accredited hospitals continues to grow. Check the Web site regularly if you're a frequent traveler.

Teaching hospitals train tomorrow's doctors by letting some of them doctor you now. One tip? If possible, try not to use a teaching hospital during the summer months. After the academic year begins in July, a new crop of fresh, green medical students and residents fills the hospital corridors. Just as you wouldn't want to have your transmission be the first ever repaired by a particular mechanic, you probably don't want to be the first patient for a med student or resident. Let them learn the basics for a few months before you become their next lesson. At the very least, you may wish to stay out of the hospital the first and second weeks in July if you can help it. Those are their first days on the job.

Finding the ER of Your Dreams

When that sudden, unpredictable, out-of-the blue bomb drops on you, and you find yourself rushing to a hospital emergency room to save your own life or a relative's or friend's, you'll be darn glad you read this chapter. As a Smart Patient, you'll know where to go and why you chose that emergency room (or emergency *department*, as the professionals there call it, but the TV show *ER* has made the latter name far more popular among the general public). You'll also know how to make the ER trip as short and painless as possible, and how to remain in control throughout this grand adventure. If you've never been, the illustration on the next page will give you a glimpse of the fun that might await you.

This knowledge will be worth more to you in a pinch that you can imagine. When judging the strength of a hospital's emergency room, you're looking for different characteristics than those represented in the hospital test, and you need to know certain things that aren't yes-no answers.

You should also ask the opinion of some people in the know. Your doctor, of course, is number one. Doctors know the scoop on the local ERs, and where they'd go if their own lives were in danger. The police officer sitting next to you at the diner counter will likely be a great informant; he's been to all of the ERs within forty miles and watched them deal with everything from

Egads! Emergency Room

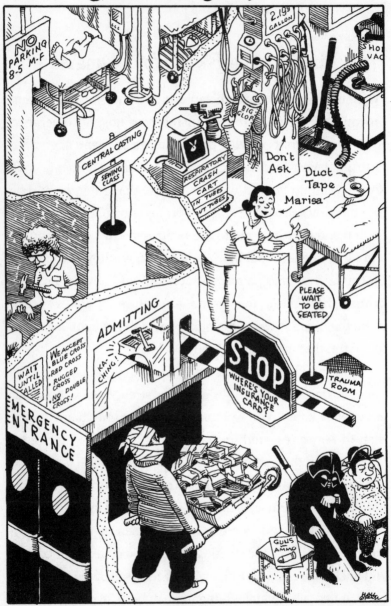

aneurysms to tent-stake impalements. Likewise, a volunteer EMT (emergency medical technician) or a county paramedic could give you an earful on which ERs are finely tuned machines and which ones he wouldn't be caught dead in. Literally.

For starters, a hospital with a great ER has to register a yes on the first three questions of the previous Smart Patient Hospital Test. If your doctor can't treat you there, your insurance won't accept, and it's not Joint Commission–accredited, that ER is the wrong choice unless it's the only choice. When is it the only choice? When it's the closest ER, and life or death depends on speed of treatment. The EMT will let you know if this is the deal. In many cases, however, it's worth driving an extra 50 minutes to a better-equipped ER than getting quicker treatment at one with fewer capabilities, believe it or not.

By the way, never drive yourself to the ER if you have heart-attack symptoms (a squeezing pain or fullness in the chest, shortness of breath, unexplained sweating, and other such symptoms; see page 186 for more details). People who try to drive themselves often never arrive. Always take an ambulance; your neighbor can't drive and defibrillate you at the same time.

When researching the ERs in your area, don't limit your search just to hospitals. Learn if there's a 24-hour urgent-care or walk-in clinic in your vicinity; going there instead can be faster and cheaper, and may be the wisest choice if the staff can handle your emergency.

What else should you ask to qualify an ER?

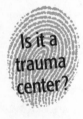

Does it have specialty docs available? One qualifying question you need to ask: Is there always a doctor on site who can open an artery in the heart or the brain, or will you have to be moved to another hospital if you need that procedure done? This is a big issue; if you're having a heart attack or a stroke, you need to go to an ER that can perform an immediate angioplasty (a procedure that opens a clogged heart artery) or a thrombolysis of a cerebral occlusion (a procedure that opens a blocked brain artery) within one hour, as this might save your life. The emergency-department nurse manager or the hospital's information line can tell you this.

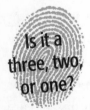

Is it a trauma center? Find out where the closest trauma center is, since that ER will be best qualified to handle injuries from auto accidents, falls, or other incidents. It's usually worth driving farther to a trauma center in these circumstances.

Is it a three, two, or one? The next thing you need to find out is an ER's level. We bet you didn't know all ERs have a level number. Level 3 ERs are tops; they have specialists and high technology at the ready and are equipped to handle anything, most notably trauma. You'll be lucky to live near (or have your accident near) a level 3 ER, and it'll probably be your best choice. ERs that rate a level 1 or 2 have a narrower repertoire and fewer specialists.

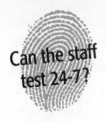

Can the staff test 24-7?

Ask if they offer round-the-clock diagnostic tests such as ultrasound, CT scans, and MRIs. You want to get these tests without delay in certain emergencies.

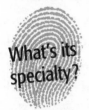

What's its specialty?

A level 1 or 2 ER may be the best choice if an emergency hits its strengths (say, if the department has a neurosurgeon, and a patient comes in with a head injury) and if a level 3 isn't anywhere in the vicinity. So learn the specific conditions that the local level 1 or 2 ERs excel in. One call to the ER nurse manager can answer that.

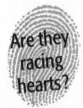

Are they racing hearts?

While you have her on the phone, find out how fast the ER treats heart emergencies. With myocardial infarctions (heart attacks), ERs have to document their average time for getting patients through the ER and into the heart catherization laboratory. They're required to make this info available, so ask for their time. How does the ER meet national benchmarks for the basics, such as giving aspirin on arrival and beta-blocking drugs within twenty-four hours to heart-attack patients? This info is also available on the Joint Commission's Web site at **www.qualitycheck.org.**

What's the wait?

Ask about the ER's average patient wait, which could be a telling figure. Obviously, in an emergency, you want to get in as fast as possible, so the hospital with the shortest average wait might be the best choice if other quality measurements are equal. You'll usually wait two to six hours at a teaching hospital ER before being treated for non-life-or-death emergencies, according to data. For a possible heart attack or stroke, you might get quicker treatment at a large teaching hospital than at a smaller community hospital if you have a choice. And if you show up at an emergency department with a problem that's obviously not an emergency—which many people do—there will probably be a race between what comes first: your name being called or the next Ice Age.

Are the ER doctors board certified in emergency medicine?

To find this out, ask the ER nurse manager. Or check with the American Board of Medical Specialties (at **www.abms.org** or 866-ASK-ABMS) and the American Board of Emergency Medicine (at **www.abem.org** or 517-332-4800, extension 381).

Is the staff skilled in pediatrics?

The best ER for you may not be the best ER for the rugrats in your life. Find out if the hospital has specific pediatric equipment and the trained pediatricians to use it. A separate treatment area for children—preferably away from the drunk stabbing victims, if convenient—counts as a big plus.

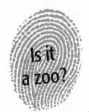

Does it like to go plastic? It's not the easiest thing to find out, but you want to ascertain from the nurse manager or another savvy source how inclined the ER docs are to call in a plastic surgeon to do some potentially tricky work, versus just doing it themselves. This isn't a life-or-death matter, but it could be a scar-or-no-scar matter. You ideally want a level 3 ER that won't hesitate to call a plastic surgeon at 2:00 A.M., versus one that will rarely reach out to a specialist.

Is it a zoo? Be a sharp detective and perform a little surveillance. Drive by the ER or poke your head in whenever you have a convenient chance in the evening or early in the morning (say, 11:00 P.M. or 7:00 A.M.). Is the line of victims snaking out the door and down the block? Are the ambulances honking furiously while bottlenecked in the driveway entrance? Look for clues of chaos and signs of organization. Two ERs with similar credentials and capabilities may be wholly different when you show up at the door, and an emergency is a lousy time to learn that you picked the one

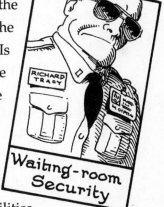

Waiting-room Security

that's a mess. Don't swing by at 3:00 P.M. to check out the ER; every ER is at its best when doctors' offices are open and handling half the would-be walk-ins.

DO THIS TODAY

Well, this week, anyway. Each of these Smart Patient moves will take you only between five seconds and twenty minutes to complete, and they could prevent the premature tapping of your life insurance by a spouse who might be spoiled by the riches.

☐ Put the Poison Control Center number on the phone.

☐ Call your police nonemergency number and check that 911 works in your area.

☐ Teach your young child to dial 911 and when to dial it.

☐ Head to a copy shop (or commandeer the work copier on the QT), copy **Your Health Journal** in appendix 2 and reduce it to its smallest readable size. Right before stashing it in your wallet, write or highlight any allergies you have (especially to drugs, rubber, or latex), and print a to-do note on it: "In an emergency, I'd like to be taken to a specific hospital, at that hospital's full address if going to this ER is practical."

☐ Right now (yes, now) read your health-insurance policy and write down exactly what you need to do when going to the ER, so you won't void your insurance. Being stuck with a $17,000 bill because your husband didn't make a phone call can dampen the euphoria of cheating death. For more specs on this, see chapter 10.

☐ Parents should consider keeping a consent form on file with the local ER. If your child has a medical emergency while you are out of town or otherwise unreachable, a consent form will allow doctors to get right to work without having to deal with the red tape of trying to obtain a social worker or court approval before giving medical assistance. If you do not feel comfortable with such a blanket consent form, you may want to discuss options with your lawyer. Your kids' school should also have a copy of the form on file in the nurse's office.

☐ If you're older than fifty, make a reduced-size copy of your last electrocardiogram test (your EKG) from your last physical, date it, and keep that in your wallet. This can save the ER staff precious time in determining how abnormally your heart is functioning compared with your usual baseline function.

☐ Put all of your medications in one place and in the original bottles, so you or someone else can grab them in an instant. Make sure that your family members or others who might be a help to you in an emergency know where your meds are.

☐ If you have a serious medical condition, such as diabetes or high blood pressure, ask your doctor if you'd be smart to wear a MedicAlert emblem or bracelet.

Just Dropping By...

Because you are a Smart Patient, we know *you know* when to visit the folks at the hospital emergency room. Why can't we have another sixty million people like you? Studies have found that more than half of all ER visits are unnecessary. This hurts two ways:

(1) The guy in front of you who's at the ER for his sinusitis is making you wait, and the triage nurse has to assess him before she can get to you. And if he talks a good game, he may convince her to let him keep his slot ahead of you.

(2) When that guy gets a $9,000 bill for abusing the ER, he might default on it, which means you'll pay more for health insurance and any services at the hospital. (Subliminal message: Do not be the guy with sinusitis in the waiting room.)

Other Patients

What are no-brainer ER situations? When you're having heart-attack symptoms, don't deliberate. If you have chest, neck, or arm pain and/or shortness of breath and/or it feels as if an elephant is sitting on your chest and/or you have indigestion plus one of the other symptoms, call the ambulance. *Now.* Signs of a stroke (that is, loss of function or prolonged numbness on one side of body) are also no-brainer signals to call an ambulance. So is bleeding like a Texas oil gusher.

You know, major things like that.

What doesn't require a trip to the ER? A sprained ankle. A flu you caught this afternoon. Lower back pain you've had for six months. A paper cut.

Checklist: How to Go to the ER . . . and Come Back

Here's the complete plan to get in, get care, get well, and get out of the ER with the least amount of abject misery possible. If you can't hold a pen because of the emergency, get someone else to tick off this checklist. The moment you've decided to go to the ER and have called 911, make sure you:

☐ Phone your primary-care doctor no matter what time of day or night. Tell your doctor the situation and ask him or her to call the ER, or even better, meet you there. Having a doctor involved will get you treated much faster.

☐ Call the ER yourself if you can't reach your doctor quickly. Or have someone else do it. You'll have an advantage if they're expecting you.

☐ Grab all of your medications—the ones you keep highly grabbable for just this purpose. Give them to the EMTs when they arrive and make sure they take them to the hospital with you.

☐ Have someone call your insurance company. It's a pain, but it's the world we live in. For more on this issue, see the sidebar "Forget About Finding My Arm, Just Call the Claims Hotline!" in chapter 10 on page 327.

☐ Focus on your main troubling symptoms when you're talking to the triage nurse. Tell the nurse about your chest pain in the last two hours. Be as specific as you can because she has the power to rocket you into the treatment room. Don't tell her that you've had ankle pain on and off for the last twelve years; that could keep you in the waiting room for the next twelve years. We're not telling you to lie; we're just telling you not to overburden the triage nurse with info that will keep you in the plastic chair next to the vending machine until well past dawn.

☐ Speaking of the plastic chair, that's the one you want. Avoid waiting-room chairs that have cloth upholstery, because they're harder to clean and . . . we trust you know where we're going with this.

☐ Don't skip any current symptoms. Mention everything, even the minor ones that you don't think are symptoms, such as sweating and anxiety, if they came on at about the same time.

☐ Tell the nurse about all of your medical conditions. Saying, "I have severe dizziness," is serious; saying, "I have severe dizziness, and I'm a diabetic," is critical. Once you make it into the examination area, ask to see the attending physician if you feel that a crisis is brewing. The first person you see may be a physician's assistant (PA) and talking directly to the attending doctor can be helpful if you feel you're not being heard. Don't just demand to see the attending doctor for the heck of it, however. And don't hesitate to let a physician's assistant stitch you; he's probably just as practiced at it (if not more) than the attending doc is.

☐ Give the attending physician **Your Health Journal**, EKG copy, and your prescription medications.

☐ With any luck, you'll be on your way home well before the next shift change. But if you're admitted, why, then the fun is just beginning. In the next chapter, we'll give you the Smart Patient tips to make sure your hospital stay is a short, healthy trip.

Want Some Click Answers?

These Web sites are great resources for finding hospitals and for finding out any incriminating details about them too. Smart Patients know them well.

Joint Commission on Accreditation of Healthcare Organizations (JCAHO)
www.qualitycheck.org
Check on hospitals by plugging in your zip code or the hospital's name.

American Hospital Association
www.aha.org/cgi-bin/mqinterconnect
Find hospitals in any location on this site.

Hospital Compare
www.hospitalcompare.hhs.gov
How did a hospital fare on treating the big three: heart attacks, heart failure, and pneumonia? Find out here.

Leapfrog Group
www.leapfroggroup.org
We mentioned this site in chapter 3, but it's also a good resource for finding a hospital. Use the search-and-compare option to rate specific hospitals.

Press Ganey Compass Awards

www.pressganey.org

This firm provides benchmark measurements for 40 percent of all U.S. hospitals that have more than one hundred beds. See which hospitals in your area received Press Ganey Compass Awards for superior performance.

HealthGrades

www.healthgrades.com

This private site rates hospitals by their diagnosis and treatment performances.

Directory of America's Hospitals

www.usnews.com/usnews/health/hospitals/hosp_home.htm

Every year *U.S. News & World Report* magazine ranks hospitals by a number of criteria; see who's on top now.

6

Have a Happily Humdrum Hospital Stay

Only $2,900 a Night and Free Sponge Baths— What a Deal! Just Make Sure You Check Out...

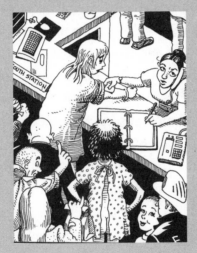

Most of us don't want to be shortchanged. We don't want to fall short of our goals, or be short on cash, time, sleep, stature, or anything else, for that matter. Boring? That's another attribute that few of us shoot for, regardless if we're talking about choosing a mate, a restaurant, or a movie.

But in a hospital, both of those qualities mean exactly one thing: pure bliss.

No matter what path you've taken to become a hospital's newest live-in guest, you want the stay to be as short and sweet as possible. Failing sweet, incredibly boring will do just fine. Boring means you didn't have any thrilling, life-threatening complications. Short and boring means things were planned well. And boring and short means you'll spend the least amount of time possible in what can be one of the most dangerous places you'll ever enter.

To put it bluntly, the hospital that helps you heal can also accidentally injure or kill you. The measures that the staffers take to care for you and the environment that caring for sick patients creates expose you to dangers that you'd never, ever face in your day-to-day life. The fact that you're usually in your weakest and most susceptible condition when you're in a hospital makes matters much worse.

The numbers? They're scary. We've already told you that as many as 98,000 patients die every year from hospital errors. Another two million hospital patients get an infection. As we said in the introduction, your personal odds of having a significant unexpected complication (meaning one that could lay you up for weeks, leave you permanently disabled, or kill you) when you check into the hospital are 1 in 25. Since you'll likely enjoy more than a few hospital trips in your lifetime, as almost all of us will, that risk will multiply.

Now, to be fair to our noble profession, there's another side to these terrifying numbers that we rarely see, and that's how many patients are healed without a hitch. It would be nice to see front-page newspaper articles screaming, "U.S.

hospitals safely treated 12 million patients this year—and directly saved the lives of at least a third!" But, to quote a famous journalism adage, newspapers don't write stories about planes that land. We all expect safety, cleanliness, and overall excellent care when we check into a hospital. And we have a right to expect it. The trouble is, the shoulds don't always match reality, for many reasons we'll explain. But they can. When you're an inpatient, you can keep a sharp eye out for the troubles that might strike you during the course of normal care.

What are those perils? They come in threes: The hospital might *infect, inject,* or *neglect* you (of course, not deliberately).

Infect? The most powerful and malicious germs you'll ever encounter—at least without burrowing through a rain forest in Tasmania— live in hospitals. You need to pay special attention to the hygiene and cleanliness of the hospital—and dirt can give you a lot of clues, as janitor-detective Easy Rawlins from *Devil in a Blue Dress* would tell you. Health care workers take extreme measures to stop these germs from hurting you, but their efforts can be sabotaged in a hundred tiny ways hundreds of times a day. Always choose a hospital with plenty of sinks and soap and/or hand-gel

Easy Rawlins

dispensers—and watch for whether they are being used . . . regularly.

Of course, patients endlessly contaminate themselves too; don't touch your wound or IV, especially after you just sneezed. Remember that you are super susceptible to germs now that you're an inpatient (not to be confused with *impatient*). Do everything you can to prevent infections from laying you low; it's one of your greatest risks while in the hospital.

Inject? We're using the broader definition of inject, meaning "to introduce into," rather than the needle-only connotation it has in medical circles, since another word wouldn't rhyme as nicely with *infect* and *neglect*. If possible, choose a hospital that tracks by using medication bar codes and your wristband and makes sure they correspond. That lessens the opportunity for the wrong drug or the wrong dosage to lengthen your stay. Great hospitals now have systems that check every syringe, IV, pill, balm, and inhaler.

Neglect? No hospital would intentionally neglect a patient, of course. (Well, except maybe the hospital depicted on the opposite page). But to call hospitals busy places is a bit like calling Texas warm and spacious. They're also full of fallible humans. Things get overlooked when they shouldn't. A nurse or doctor may do ninety-nine things per-

Oh, No, I Won't Go to the Hospital Room

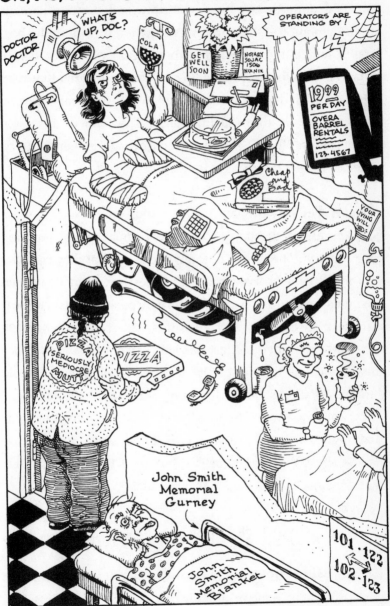

fectly but forget about the 100th. And once in a great while, that 100th item can be a big deal. Knowing this, Smart Patients are not among the shy and reserved when they're in the hospital. If something seems amiss, they speak up. So should you. In fact, if you see hospital staffers wearing buttons that read "Speak Up!" it doesn't mean they blew out their eardrums by standing too close to the fire alarm. The Joint Commission gives staffers these buttons to encourage patients to be squeaky wheels.

Smart Patients prepare for a hospital stay with the same focus and dedication to details as combat pilots preparing for a mission. They leave nothing to chance that they can control and accept no risk that isn't necessary. They've chosen hospitals as carefully as a flying ace inspects his plane. Pilots also keep in close contact with their ground crew, because they know that their biggest risk isn't catching a surface-to-air missile through the cockpit; it's a loose bolt on their tail hook.

Smart Patients are the top guns of health care consumers. They know to sweat the small stuff—meaning the elements that might *seem* small, such as a doctor not washing his or her hands before touching your IV—but are actually the dangers that are most likely to cause real trouble.

Just Swallowing Orders

We've already discussed the perils of medication errors, so you know how dangerous they can be. But in the hospital, you need to multiply that danger many times. You're probably going to have a conga line of staffers giving you strange pills and IV meds around the clock, and you'll be one of twenty-five people they're going past as they dispense their goods. These people will constantly change, and each will attempt to follow constantly changing medication orders from several different doctors who are treating you.

It's easy to see how drug mistakes kill at least 40,000 and maybe 80,000 hospital patients every year. To avoid joining them, use this defense:

Pick one doctor to head the team

To shorten your stay, you want one doctor to act as the head coach, calling (or approving) all the signals, and you want that doctor to be on the job full time. Have your primary-care doctor lead the team if she's able to spend enough time in the hospital with you. Or have one hospitalist (a full-time hospital doctor without a private practice) who knows your primary-care doc well coordinate everything.

Or you could ask your specialist if he or she has the time to oversee all of your care. You want one doctor to oversee your entire

Specialist

treatment regimen, approve all prescriptions, and know everything that's going on. This will help avoid mistakes and also help you get the heck out of that hospital as soon as possible.

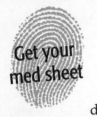

Ask your doctor or nurse to give you a copy of your medication administration record, which will list all of the drugs you're supposed to take (at least as of that moment), and their dosages and frequencies. Don't be too embarrassed to ask for this. (This is a great job for your advocate too.)

Go over the list with your doctor and nurses to find out why you need each drug, and what kinds of effects you might expect after taking it. Whenever someone gives you medication of any sort, check it against your med sheet.

Ask the nurse to double-check your wrist identification band during every pill offering to be certain you're the right patient. Actually, a hospital accredited by the Joint Commission is required to get two patient identifiers (for example, your name and Social Security number) every time staff members give you a drug, draw blood, or wheel you away for a test. They should not be taking the sloppy shortcut of using your room number or bed number as your identifier; that's inviting error, because patients move around.

Make sure your drug allergies are mentioned on that band, in case you can't speak up for yourself. Once again, choosing a hospital that uses bar-code readers to match prescriptions against a bar code on your wrist ID band can save a lot of worry.

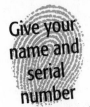

Don't just let the nurse scan or read silently to check your identity; verbally tell him or her your full name and the last four digits of your Social Security number to make sure they jibe with the paperwork. This is a smart safeguard against mistakes, as nurses can find themselves—as the illustration on page 203 shows—a little busy at times, to say the least.

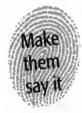

After they check your ID band and verbally confirm your name and last four Social Security digits, politely ask them to tell you what they're giving you and why. A nice way to say it: "Could you please refresh me on what this drug is and what it does?" If that checks, recite your drug allergies, even if your ID band blares them. Then you should be good to gulp.

THE SLEEPWALKING SOCIETY

You've seen enough television shows and heard enough horror stories to know that doctors and nurses routinely work more hours without a break than most accountants in April. And working such hours isn't an unusual once-in-a-while occurrence. It's a tribute to the backup and safety systems and to their intelligence and diligence that the error rates aren't ten times as great, given how overextended and sleep deprived many hospital staffers are. And let's not even talk about the extra challenges of the night shift. Nurses who work longer than twelve-hour shifts or more than forty hours a week are three times more likely to make medical errors. More than half of these errors involve medication.

Resident doctors envy these nurses for all the sack time they get, because many starting doctors work an average of 105 hours a week. To stop or at least reduce some of that madness, the Accreditation Council for Graduate Medical Education (which accredits 7,800 residency programs in the United States) ruled that residents must not work more than 80 hours in a week or more than 24 hours in a row. In addition, they must get one day off per week.

Generous, huh? Well, it helped; in hospitals without restrictions, resident hours have dropped to 74 hours a week from 105 hours a week. Not a typo. If new doctors were forced to work only 13 hours a day for six days straight, many would feel like they'd gone part-time.

A Shifty Situation

Be especially watchful during and right after shift changes; they're the most treacherous time for mistakes. Aside from jibing with common sense, it's been proven: a study published in the *British Medical Journal* in 2001 found that babies born at

Nerves of Steel Nurse Station

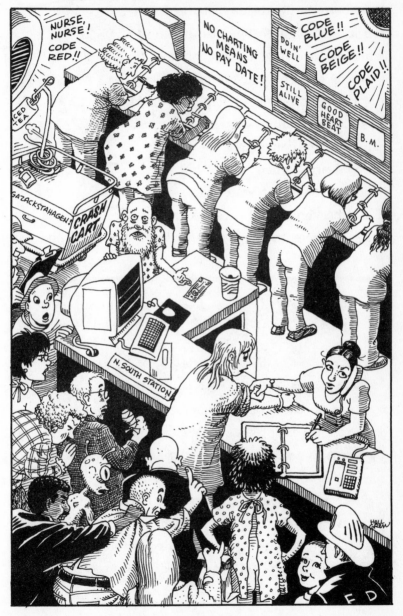

night had a greater risk of dying than babies born during the day; but babies born around shift change also had a higher risk of dying. The cacophony of coming and going, the transfer of info, the handing off of half-done tasks—it's not hard to see why shift changes up the danger ante.

So learn when the shift changes take place in your hospital and be vigilant. Always ask the nurse, "Is there anything specific that I should tell the

Staff Nurse

BE A SMART (AND GRATEFUL) PATIENT

Keep a candy dish in your room for the nurses, and stock it with good stuff. Chocolate is always popular. Ordering a couple of large pizzas for the nurses at lunch or dinnertime to show your appreciation isn't a bad idea, either, because they often miss their meals. And it goes without saying that you should learn each nurse's name, and preferably her children's hobbies and talents. Make a note of it if you have to. If you've never been a people person in your life, now is a good time to get good at it. Saying please and thank you and treating nurses and other staff as respectfully and kindly as possible would be a great thank-you, as would writing the hospital CEO a note extolling the great nursing care.

next nurse after you guys do the shift-change staff report?" In part, you're really asking, "What should *you* tell your replacement so nothing happens to me?" Don't get us wrong: nurses are the most compassionate, smart people we know, and they fight for you. But they get overworked too, so giving them reminders never hurts.

Declare Germ Warfare

The biggest enemy you have in the hospital isn't your phone-addicted roommate. It's much smaller. And there are billions of them. They have names like *B staphylococcus* (or staph), *Klebsiella,* and *enterobacter.* One may have even visited you before; his name is *E coli.* He's responsible for half of all hospital infections. You've no doubt read some interesting stories about *Streptococcus pyogenes,* whose nickname is "flesh-eating bacteria." Of the 2 million hospital infections reported yearly, he has a hand in only about 15,000.

Many bugs like these live on us, in us, or with us every day, harmlessly. In fact, there's a constant *War of the Worlds* going on inside you every moment with good bacteria relentlessly preventing bad bacteria from multiplying too plentifully. Other, more bizarre varieties congregate only in places hoarded with sick people 365 days a year, namely hospitals. When they get into new territory, like a wound, or your lung, or your heart, some begin attacking you ferociously. Those bugs are normally easy prey for your immune system's killer cells. But now they find you defenseless, since your illness has already plundered your body's defenses.

These hospital infections cause 90,000 deaths annually and add an average of two weeks to hospital stays, according to research published in the *New England Journal of Medicine*. The most crucial tip you need to follow to prevent a hospital infection is one you've heard before. One that's constantly ignored or forgotten. And one that Smart Patients take as seriously as monitoring the drugs they swallow and choosing the surgeons who try to repair them. It can be distilled to three clear words:

Wash Your Hands!

This order goes to every single person who may come in contact with you. They need to scrub their paws. Before touching you. Before touching your sheets, or your water cup, or your side table, or anything else that you could conceivably touch. If they're conscientious enough to put on new rubber gloves as well, that would be marvelous. But hand washing is mandatory. This is not a joke. They should wash their hands after they touch you and before they head to the next patient.

It's understandable that harried nurses and doctors occasionally forget to do this, but it's not acceptable. No hospital should have a room without a sink or an alcohol hand-gel dispenser. No clinic or doctor's office either. Posting a sign in your room that says, THANKS VERY MUCH FOR WASHING YOUR HANDS, can help. This goes for all visitors, and for you too.

If you're able to get up, wash your hands with soap and water several times a day (especially after you hug or shake hands with a visitor). Don't just do a three-second rinse; the helpful folks at the Centers for Disease Control and Prevention (CDC) say you need to wash vigorously for at least fifteen seconds with soap and warm water (about the time it takes to sing "Happy Birthday," the alphabet song, or "I wish I were an Oscar Mayer Wiener"), hitting your palms, the backs of your hands, and between your fingers. You could alternatively use an alcohol sanitizing gel, which will obviously be easier if you're not mobile.

The importance of hand washing to prevent infection is such a big deal that the Joint Commission came up with buttons for nurses, doctors, and other health care staff to wear that read: ASK ME IF I'VE WASHED MY HANDS. So, if you see those on your health care givers' lab coats (or even if you don't), ask away. Don't be shy about it. Unlike the sarcastic bumper stickers that read, HOW'S MY DRIVING? DIAL . . . , these buttons are meant to be taken a tad more seriously.

By the way, you know you should wash your hands frequently to avoid colds and other transmissible nuisances every day *outside* the hospital too, so here's a money-saving (and perhaps humanity-saving) tip: don't use antibacterial soap. The Food and Drug Administration found that antibacterial soap doesn't clean your hands any better than plain ol' soap. And, like unnecessary antibiotics, it helps create bacteria strains that are harder to kill.

Other tips to reduce the odds of infection:

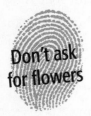

Your first gift should be an industrial-sized jug of alcohol hand-sanitizing gel, as recommended before. Keep it by your bed and ask all visitors who might conceivably touch you (even for a conjugal visit) to help themselves to a generous dollop. Yes, the hospital will supply disinfectant to your room, but for less than $20 you can remind every staff person how important this measure is to you—and offer an attention-getting backup to the ubiquitous jug of hospital disinfectant that tends to blend in with the wallpaper for hospital workers after they treat a few thousand patients.

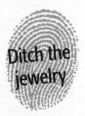

Your wedding ring isn't only at risk of being lost or stolen, or becoming a bullet if accidentally taken into an MRI tube (depending on what metal it's made of, though this is a really bad way to find out), but it's a germ trap. Don't take it with you to the hospital. And the nose ring, Forget it. We're not even allowed to wear them in the ER.

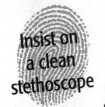

Don't touch your IV or surgical site even with freshly washed hands. It should be covered with a sterile barrier, but don't trust it. Wash your hands especially thoroughly before sleeping because you're liable to touch surgical and IV sites accidentally. And wash every time you get up at night, as germs will migrate back to your hands.

Ask for a tube that's coated with an antiseptic Contaminated catheters used to draw blood or supply nutrients or medications cause about 250,000 patient infections every year. Researchers at the University of Nebraska Medical Center found that using antiseptic-coated catheters—and being extra careful to maintain the catheter's sterility—can greatly lower your odds of picking up an infection this way.

Insist on a clean stethoscope Stethoscopes are filthy from being used on several patients an hour without being cleaned at all or having a new rubber barrier put on. Most docs now wash their stethoscopes with alcohol between patients, but we'd always ask. To keep things light, be a humorist. Say, "I'm taking a survey; did you wash that stethoscope with alcohol or soap and water?"

Keep it secure

If you have a wound dressing, a catheter, or a drainage tube, tell a nurse if it becomes wet or loose.

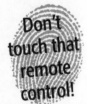

Treat the bathroom like the bus station restroom

Namely, don't touch the toilet lever or especially the faucet handle; that's the last thing the nurse touched after treating the highly infectious guy next door. If you must touch it (elbows and knees count), disinfect the area with an alcohol gel. Or use a clean paper towel to turn the faucet off.

Don't touch that remote control!

Or wear rubber gloves if you want to click through the daytime soaps. A study found that the television remote control is one of the most germ-infested things in a hospital room. The remotes had more than three times as much bacteria as the room doorknobs, the nurse

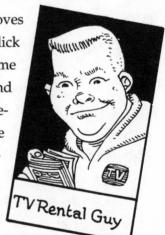

TV Rental Guy

call button, and the tray table. Many of those bugs were lethal killers. And you thought the TV could just bore you to death.

Disposable remote controls meant for short use were far

cleaner, so grab one of them if there's a choice. Cleaning the remote control with small dabs of the disinfectant gel is another option.

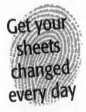

Get your sheets changed every day

And ask for a new disposable pillow when you check into your room. We realize this might feel environmentally irresponsible to you, since that's the reason hospitals (and hotels) cite for changing sheets less frequently, in addition to cost and staffing shortages. How about this: be regretfully environmentally irresponsible while in the hospital by getting new sheets and pillows every day, and then volunteer for an environmental organization after you check out infection free. You'll do more good alive.

Ask them to send their love via phone

Visitors are nice, but they're also cargo ships full of bacteria. They touch things they're not supposed to. They pour water with your jug and hand you the cup. They bring flowers and cards in envelopes they licked. They let the kids hop up on the bed. They kiss you. Everyone feels better to see you feeling better.

That visit may have just added another two weeks to your stay if you get an infection from the bugs they left with you.

Hey, we love visitors when we're sick, too. We're just telling you the trade-off. Have them phone. You remember what they look like, right?

We'd keep visitors to a minimum, or make sure they scrub

up and keep their hands in their pockets when they come see you. Tell them your docs insist on this, if you need to make us the bad guys. We're used to it.

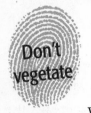

Don't vegetate

Get up and start moving around as soon as you can. In fact, practice every day for at least one week before elective surgery. We've found with our own patients that a week of daily walking prior to an operation can help people recover significantly faster. It's especially important after a procedure; thousands of patients every year are infected with pneumonia because they don't move enough. Walking helps your lungs get rid of bacteria-infested mucus. Of course, check with your doctor or nurse before you hop out of bed and start trotting off to parts unknown. Be sure you're ready and have someone accompany you during the first few outings. This is one of the most important tips you can take, so write yourself a note if necessary.

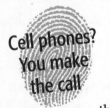

Cell phones? You make the call

Keeping in touch with your health care team is often a challenge when you're in the hospital, since if you're not unconscious, asleep, or being sewn, kneaded, or wheeled about by the staff, you're able to make calls only via the expensive room phone. And your family members and health care advocate are also hamstrung, because they can't use their cell phones in the hospital, according to the official policies. To

be honest, we've seen plenty of visitors and patients ignoring said policies;
it depends on the hospital.

However, as a Smart (and oh-so-
discreet) Patient, you can probably obtain
permission to use a cell phone in your room
or the rest room without worrying about
short-circuiting a patient's ventilator down the
hall. Research published in the medical journal
Mayo Clinic Proceedings found that cell phones posed
little danger to the functioning of hospital medical devices. In
a test, they affected function in only about 1.2 percent of cases
and had no effect at all on half the machines tested. So if it becomes an issue, kindly tell the nurses what the Mayo Clinic
found. And make sure you wipe down that germy cell phone
with disinfectant before you use it.

It Takes Two

Smart Hospital Patients adhere to the same rule number one
as mountain climbers, scuba divers, and kindergarteners on
field trips: Never do it alone. Buddy up! You need a trusted
friend or family member to stick by you—both literally and
figuratively—and act as your health care advocate, which we
defined back in chapter 3 on page 102. Once again, think of
this person as your partner: the Thelma to your Louise, the
Butch Cassidy to your Sundance Kid (although your adven-

ture will end more pleasantly than theirs, for sure). He or she will take notes during doctor's visits, ask questions that you may have overlooked, and act as your essential cover-your-back person to ensure that your doctors and nurses—and you—follow the tips in this book. Your advocate can make phone calls, check on tests, nudge people, and solve problems while you rest or concentrate on rehabilitating. She will shorten your stay. (Sorry, guys, but 80 percent of advocates are women.)

Although she won't have legal authority to make decisions for you unless you specifically give it to her (we'll tell you when that may be in your best interest in chapter 8), let the hospital staff know that your advocate is a card-carrying member of your health care team, not just a concerned friend or relative, and certainly not an adversary. Tip: treat your advocate that way, and the staff will too.

As with choosing a great hospital, you should choose your health care advocate before you need one. Who can you tap? A willing friend or relative with a medical background is a great choice, but your advocate doesn't have to be an expert—just dedicated.

Aside from having enough time to do this job, she also needs to have the right temperament for it. You'll need to work together well. Be careful about picking the most convenient person if she's clearly not up to the job. Just as you wouldn't deputize the first cousin you meet in the family-reunion buffet line, don't automatically pick your spouse just because he or she is nearby, especially if he or she also happens to be terrified of blood or is the most disorganized person you know. Someone who's extremely stressed and anguished by needlesticks might make a poor advocate because you need someone who's going to stay objective. A Smart Patient finds an advocate who will stay cool and clear minded in a crisis.

Did Someone Make You Spew Profanity?

The hospital wasn't clean, or your meds were consistently screwed up? The place just isn't safe? Get mad! Complain! Here's how:

If you're in a Joint Commission–accredited hospital (another reason to choose one), voice your grievance (anonymously, if you prefer) by calling the Joint Commission's Complaint Line at 800-994-6610 (weekdays, 8:30 A.M. to 5:00 P.M. central time). Or describe the problem in no more than two pages and e-mail it to **complaint@jcaho.org.** You can also find the form at **www.jcaho.org**; click on "General Public," then click on "Go to Report a Complaint." You can fill it out online or print it out and mail it to the address given on the Web site. Make sure you include all the identifying information about the health care organization (name, full address, city, and state).

If the patient is still in the offending hospital, or you're an employee there, don't worry about retaliation, because it's kept strictly confidential (honestly). What can't the Joint Commission help you with? Billing issues or disputes, insurance issues, personnel concerns, and anything at all at an unaccredited facility. Call if you're in doubt.

Be It Ever So Humble

Discharge time?

Excellent! You made it.

A hospital stay is a surefire way to bring out the inner Dorothy in all of us; however magical the journey, the thought of going home grows sweeter every day. Smart Patients don't just look forward to going home, they prepare for it—whether they're in the hospital for two days or two months. Given that 1 in 5 hospital patients undergoing major procedures suffer a significant complication after returning home, it's wise to make a careful reentry plan.

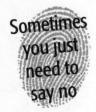

Sometimes you just need to say no

As eager as you are to get out of the hospital—and we know you'd never hang around the place as if it were a spa—sometimes you may not be physically ready to go home when the hospital (or your health-insurance company) wants to discharge you. However great the temptation to leave, you can put yourself in danger or experience a new high in misery if you head home while still needing hospital care. Ask your doctor to extend your stay, and if that doesn't work, "escalate the situation," as they say in customer service. Enlist your advocate. Ask the department's head doctor for help, call your insurance company, and otherwise go up the chain until you're ringing 1600 Pennsylvania Avenue.

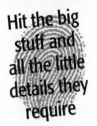 **Hit the big stuff and all the little details they require** Think of all the tasks you'll need done after going home and what they'll entail. With your advocate and family's help, make a to-do list, give each item a deadline, then parcel out the duties. Or entrust someone to oversee this for you, if necessary. For example, if you'll need a nurse or therapist to treat you at home, ask your advocate to help you get recommendations for a home health care company. (By the way, the Joint Commission accredits home health care agencies too.) Have her clear it with your insurer and set up the appointments.

Make sure you have enough supplies on hand. Arrange help with cooking, cleaning, shopping, and getting to and from the doctor's office. If you need to set up a temporary bedroom on the first floor to avoid stairs, have it ready before you get home. If you'll be taking medicine at home, get the prescription filled at the hospital outpatient pharmacy before you leave. People tend to navigate hospital adventures day by day and don't think of these things until the last minute. That causes all sorts of headaches.

Find out who you should call

Don't just assume you'll call your doctor for any problem; there may be a better person or a faster person to reach. Ask your surgeon and your primary-care doctor who you should contact with any follow-up issues or problems involving medication, pain, bleeding, fever, questions about take-home equipment, catheters, and the like. Everyone forgets to ask this, and it can be one of the most important points of information you get.

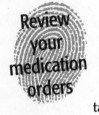

Review your medication orders

If you'll be taking any meds or written prescriptions at home, ask the doctor or nurse to explain what each one is, what it does, why you need to take it, when and how you should take it, and when you can stop taking it. Also ask about the drugs you took before you went into the hospital and if any of the new ones substitute for these, or if you should take these. Importantly, you may be taking home the hospital's version of another drug you already have at home, even though the pills look nothing alike and have completely different names. You don't want to mistakenly take both.

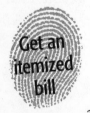

Get an itemized bill

Not before discharge, but before you pay. If any questions arise, make an appointment to go over it with the hospital's patient-billing advocate. Hunt for mistakes, overcharges, and any other costly gaffe. The bill will be riddled with indecipherable jargon and acronyms, although the large monetary figures will be clear. You'll need help translating it, and your insurance company may not offer it. If you're footing 20 percent of the total, you don't want to be charged twice for a $1,700 test. (And you don't want your insurance company to be charged twice; it ups everyone's rate.)

Checklist: Debrief the Doc

Make sure you review your discharge plan with both your in-hospital physician (who's either a hospitalist, a specialist, or your surgeon) and your primary-care doctor, so each knows the plan. Your advocate should be at your side when you ask these questions, taking copious notes or tape recording the conversation. (We don't mind that, honestly.) In addition to any specific questions relating to your case, don't forget to get answers to these essentials and to write them down:

- [ ] How can I expect to feel in the coming days?
- [ ] What kinds of danger signs or complications should I watch for? How often do these kinds of complications occur?
- [ ] If I experience pain, what should I do? What kind of pain medication can I take?
- [ ] Do I need to follow a special diet at home? Any foods to avoid? No alcohol?

☐ Will I need any outpatient therapy? What kind? How will it be scheduled?

☐ What activities should I avoid at home?

☐ When can I return to work or school?

☐ When can I drive again? How about riding my Harley Davidson?

☐ When can I resume sexual activity?

☐ Can I take a shower and/or bath when I get home?

☐ How should I care for my incision and/or dressing?

☐ Should I continue taking the medications I'm currently taking? Will I have to take any additional drugs? What are they designed to do?

☐ When can I start exercising? Are there any exercises I can do to help speed healing?

☐ When can I return to my usual workout routine?

☐ When should I return for a follow-up appointment? To whom? Any follow-up tests?

☐ If I have an urgent issue, who should I call and what should I do?

☐ If I have general recovery questions, who should I call?

WANT TO KNOW MORE?

Surf these Web sites for more info on hospital safety.

Agency for Healthcare Research and Quality
www.ahrq.gov/consumer
This site, a U.S. government agency, offers consumer information about safer health care while in the hospital.

Care pointers.com
www.carepointers.com
The site, sponsored by an independent nonprofit organization, includes information about ways to stay safe in the hospital.

Medically Induced Trauma Support Services (MITSS)
www.mitss.org
This site, sponsored by a nonprofit organization that assists people affected by medically induced trauma, includes list of resources for patients.

Hand Washing/CDC
www.cdc.gov/ncidod/op/handwashing.htm
Detailed information about why it's important to wash your hands and proper technique.

7

Why You Should Always Get a Second Opinion

Whose Life Is It, Anyway?

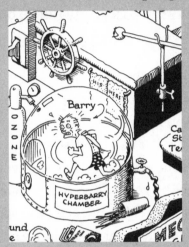

It's a two-word utterance that used to cause great tension between doctors and patients, long before "I'll sue!" stole its thunder. Mentioning it still causes anxiety, at least among a percentage of patients who can't shake their outdated notions about us doctors having some sort of all-knowing, all-seeing power.

It's "second opinion."

Of course, today we all know (or should know) the modern viewpoint on second opinions, since talk shows, nightly news segments, newspaper and magazine articles, highway billboards, health-insurance newsletters, at least a million self-help books, and everything else short of fortune cookies and *Bazooka Joe* comics have been hammering the rule into our heads for at least fifteen years:

Never Think Twice About Getting a Second Opinion

You might think that this is difficult for us to say, because, well, it boils down to admitting that we can be wrong and we can be wrong a lot. Sometimes 180 degrees wrong. But it's actually second nature for us to push second opinions. Honestly, to forget about your needs for a moment, you're doing your doctor a big favor by getting a second opinion. You're giving him the chance to have his work and his instincts checked by another qualified doctor, which can only result in three possibilities.

First, the consulting doctor could agree with his diagnosis and advice completely, which will make everyone feel more confident in going forward. Second, the consulting doctor could agree on some points but offer different thoughts on others. Third, the next opinion could be completely different. In either of the last two cases, you've given your doctor a free opportunity to learn something without him having to fly to Salt Lake City to sit through a conference. So from a purely selfless standpoint, never feel embarrassed about going for a second opinion. Your health insurance may require it in many circumstances, but even if not, your doctor almost assuredly expects you to do so. And your doctor should thank you for it. In case he or she forgets, we will:

Thanks!

Feel free to copy these pages and give them to your doctor.

Now, let's talk about the purely selfish reasons for getting a second opinion. It could save you a lot of trouble, and it could save *you*, period. No smart detective would hang his whole investigation on a single witness's story without making sure it checked out. And no Smart Patient would hang her whole life on a single expert's judgment. Research has found that getting a second opinion results in a new diagnosis in as many as 30 percent of all cases. That's a lot of cases.

Why, oh why, then, do people still regard second opinions the way they regarded psychiatry twenty-five years ago? They say it in hushed tones, as if they were talking about an upcoming lobotomy (no offense to those with upcoming lobotomies) or an illicit drug transaction. One day we expect to hear a patient spelling it out to another patient in the waiting room ("I'm getting an *S-E-C* . . ."), hoping that what keeps her three-year-old guessing will also trick us.

It would be funny, except this stigma affects decisions. Research shows that only 20 percent of people who seek medical care every year get a second opinion. If only one out of five people seek a second opinion, but almost one in three second opinions result in new diagnoses . . . The math is making our heads hurt, but the implication is obvious. There are millions of patients who aren't getting second opinions who clearly should—and doing so would change the treatment course for large numbers of them. Today, getting second opinions is easier than ever due to technologies that allow doctors to consult from afar. Just like Dick Tracy, use all the technology at your disposal to make getting a second opinion easier. Whether it's email, overnight delivery services, or a two-way spy receiver.

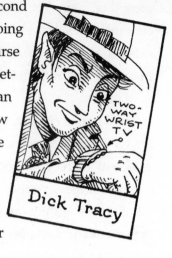

Dick Tracy

We Need a Hero

This reluctance is understandable in some ways. When you have a health crisis, there's a strong inner desire to put complete faith in your doctor, to see her as a shining beacon of leadership and serenity, a port in the storm, someone who will tell you, *"This is what we will do, and it's going to be okay."* This gives you a strong sense of clarity: *Doc says do this, so we'll do this.*

Realizing that you need a second opinion is admitting that this notion is all just a comforting fairy tale, and your doctor is not an infallible authority, but just a human being who's doing his or her best and could very well be wrong. She might've been watching a *West Wing* rerun last week instead of reading the latest medical journal that discussed a new treatment for your condition. Stripping your physician of this reassuring myth of invincibility can make you feel even more adrift and alone when you're in a bad situation.

Those are the deeper psychological roilings. The roilings right on the surface? When you say, "I'm going to get a second opinion," it's easy to feel as if you're telling your doctor that you think her medical knowledge is spotty, so you're going to find a real pro. And in talking with the second-opinion doctor, it's easy to feel that the unpleasant subtext of your questions may inch perilously close to: "This doctor that I've been trusting my life with for eleven years . . . does she really know what she's doing?"

To heck with all the psychobabble stuff. Smart Patients always get a second opinion in important situations. That's one of the biggest reasons they're Smart.

Checklist: By George, He Thinks I've Got It

If your doctor diagnoses you with any problem, get the full facts by ticking off these questions. The answers will help you decide if you need a second opinion and will also be useful to the second doctor in determining exactly where you stand.

☐ How do you know I have this condition? How was it diagnosed? Was a Ouija board involved?

- [ ] What does this condition mean for my overall health?
- [ ] Can it be treated? Does it have to be treated? What happens if I don't get it treated?
- [ ] Should you conduct further tests to confirm the diagnosis? If you do, why are those tests necessary? What kinds of side effects or risks do they involve?
- [ ] What kinds of treatment options do I have? What are the pros and cons of different treatments?
- [ ] What are the benefits of seeking a second opinion?
- [ ] How can I find out more information about this condition or disease?
- [ ] Is there anything I can do to help control the condition?
- [ ] Who is the best in the world at treating this?
- [ ] Are there any clinical trials under way for this condition or disease?
- [ ] Where would you go if you had this disease, and who would you see? Is this person the absolute best expert for this condition, and if not, why on earth would you seek him out? (You're not asking him to give you an "If I were you . . ." response, you're asking him where he'd go to protect his own life.)

Is Now the Time?

A lot of people have the perception that second opinions are only for life-and-death situations. Say, when your doctor diagnoses you with something serious, or when he wants to take your leg off (even if he's told you why). But there are plenty of common circumstances in which having another physician weigh in could be a big help. Even those as seemingly routine as managing high blood pressure, or perhaps diagnosing a persistent skin rash that your doctor thinks is harmless. Even if your life isn't at stake, feel free to seek a second opinion if:

- ☞ Your doctor says you need surgery.
- ☞ Your doctor is stumped by your condition and can't diagnose it.
- ☞ Your doctor isn't a specialist in the disease you have. You need to consult a highly qualified specialist as your second-opinion doctor— hopefully one with an office that doesn't resemble the one on page 230 too closely.

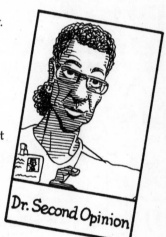

Dr. Second Opinion

- ☞ The care or treatment you're receiving just isn't working after a reasonable period of time.
- ☞ Your doctor doesn't seem to be taking your symptoms seriously enough.
- ☞ You've lost faith in your doctor, or you've ceased to communicate well with each other.

Sub-par Specialist's Office

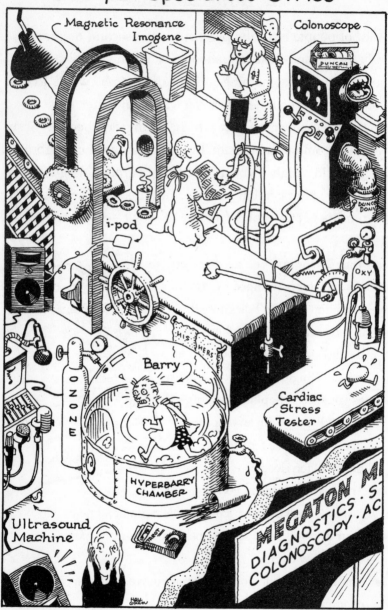

☞ You want to try other treatment options. Be careful here, because if you keep looking, you'll eventually find a doctor who will tell you what you want to hear. (See the sidebar "Don't Shoot the Messenger" on page 234.)

But Do You Have the Time?

Don't feel pressured into forgoing a second opinion if your doctor says your problem requires speedy treatment. Except in the most dire cases, which are quite rare (say, when a heart attack could happen at any second), you'll almost always have at least a few days to get a second opinion. When you call someone in hopes of getting that second opinion, make sure you tell the nurse or receptionist that you're seeking a second opinion and need to be seen quickly. Make sure you research your condition on your own, so you're as knowledgeable as possible. (We'll hit this momentarily). The peace of mind is almost always worth the time investment.

But what about the cash investment? *Just who will pay for this second opinion,* you're wondering? Most insurance plans cover second opinions because they care about you—and because it makes good financial sense. They'd rather not pay $50,000 for a heart operation when there's a chance that you need only a $3,500 preventive-medicine program. For this reason, many insurers *require* you to get a second opinion before they'll pay for certain major procedures. This is a fantastic thing for patients who'd be too sheepish to get a second opinion on their own.

Not all insurance plans are so forward thinking, sadly. If you have an HMO or managed-care plan, it may not cover a second opinion. If you can't persuade the insurer to open its wallet (more about that in chapter 10), it may be well worthwhile to pay for the second opinion out of your own pocket. Sure, this won't be cheap, but it could be the best money you'll ever spend in your life. Before you whip out your checkbook, though, read your entire policy carefully and check the laws in your state. (This is a great job for your advocate, by the way.) Some states, including California and New York, have passed laws that guarantee members of HMOs the right to get a second opinion.

What Did We Miss?

Just as the best detectives and would-be Sherlocks end up collaring the wrong suspect now and then, doctors often blame the wrong disease or condition for a patient's symptoms. Misdiagnoses aren't always the mark of a shoddy professional. Hundreds of diseases have almost exactly the same symptoms, and many others, maddeningly, have no symptoms at all until they wreak havoc.

Just how frequently do we get it wrong? It's impossible to know exactly, as records are difficult to keep, but different surveys have suggested that as many as 40 percent of all diagnoses may be wrong. Of course, doctors came up with this figure, so that could be wrong too! In truth, it's probably overblown, and the real percentage is far lower (that's our story, and we're sticking to it). But one thing is certain: misdiagnosis is an extremely common medical error. For example, a study of almost 2,500 autopsies found that almost 40 percent had at least one significant undiagnosed disease. Another autopsy study found that doctors missed a problem in one out of every four patients; and in more than two-thirds of those cases, the patients would have likely received different treatment or lived longer had their overlooked disease been found.

Which diseases do we miss most? Like the common-faced suspects who are the hardest to pick out of a police lineup, they're the maladies that have vague symptoms or hide behind other diseases, letting them wrongly take the rap. Below are common culprits. They're often missed by doctors in the initial exams and caught only in later follow-ups, many by second-opinion docs.

☛ Chronic fatigue syndrome doesn't have any specific diagnostic test.

☛ Depression can cause a variety of physical and emotional symptoms.

☛ Fibromyalgia, like chronic fatigue syndrome, can cause a wide range of symptoms.

☛ Glaucoma, which can lead to blindness, doesn't cause symptoms early on.

☛ The genetic disease hemochromatosis causes iron overload in some of the body's organs, yet has no early symptoms.

☛ High blood pressure, or hypertension, may produce no early symptoms.

- Impaired glucose tolerance and type 2 diabetes can produce mild symptoms that occur gradually.
- Kidney disease, which can be life threatening, may trigger few early symptoms.
- Osteoporosis, which causes thinning bones, is often diagnosed only after the person suffers a bone fracture.
- Polycystic ovary syndrome causes hormonal and menstrual symptoms and can lead to infertility.
- Sexually transmitted diseases such as syphilis, chlamydia, trichomoniasis, bacterial vaginosis, gonorrhea, and the human papilloma virus (HPV). These diseases may have no major symptoms, or it may take years for them to show up. Many masquerade as arthritis and dementia.
- Dementia can often be due to mercury or lead poisoning, though that cause is rarely diagnosed at first.
- Thyroid disorders, such as hypothyroidism, can cause vague symptoms like fatigue and weakness.
- Mental fogginess caused by medication overload, depression, or fluid in the brain, which many physicians wrongly attribute to Alzheimer's disease.

DON'T SHOOT THE MESSENGER

In some countries—such as Turkey, Korea, China, and Italy—ask a person how he's doing after his doctor gives him a clean bill of health, and he might reply, "Thanks for asking, I'm dying." Maybe these folks have a morbid sense of humor, but for many such a thought (well, more or less) stems from a basic lack of trust in their doctors. Simply, in their cultures, if doctors don't have anything nice to tell patients, many still believe that he should, well, lie. An old person has cancer? Don't tell her! A young person has a disease? Don't tell him what those pills are for. Why be a downer? And why risk having patients hate you because you gave them news that they didn't want to hear?

Well, in the United States we do things a little differently. We give the full truth. It's part of our creed here.

Why do we mention this? Because some patients hold a bad diagnosis against their doctor. Then they shop for a second opinion—not to increase the accuracy of their diagnosis, but simply to hear the news that they want to hear from a doctor (or alternative-medicine practitioner) who will willingly contradict their first physician.

And guess what? If they ask enough doctors and practitioners, they'll find someone who will tell them exactly what they want to hear, whether it's true or ethical or dangerous or not.

It can be difficult to give a patient bad news, and still have them respect you and believe you're doing your ultimate best to help them. So please don't shoot the messenger—or shoot yourself by searching for a second opinion to satisfy a grudge against Dr. Evil.

The 1-2-3s of Second Opinions

To get this ball rolling, your first task (or your advocate's first task) is to find a qualified, unbiased doctor who can give you the best second opinion possible. Many patients find second-opinion doctors through physician referral services, such as "DoctorFinder," offered by the American Medical Association at **www.ama-assn.org.** You can also get help through medical societies and organizations centering on specific health conditions. Can you ask your existing doctor for a few names? Sure. But we wouldn't advise going that route. That's because you ideally want to:

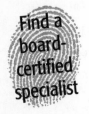

Find a board-certified specialist This can be a tall order in some circumstances, especially if your first doctor was also a specialist. But the effort to find such a physician is worthwhile. It's simple human nature: your doctor will likely recommend another physician she knows and respects, perhaps a good friend she considers the best doctor in the county. Two doctors who are friends are less likely to contradict each other.

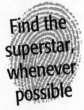

Find the superstar, whenever possible A smart lawyer wouldn't call the first impressive-sounding expert witness she found in the yellow pages to testify in court; she'd find the expert's expert. Likewise, a Smart Patient won't just find another qualified doctor when getting a second opinion. Whenever possible, he'll go to the hospital, university, or medical facility that's known for treating his particular disease and tap the most respected physician there (if he hasn't already tapped a specialist from there to be his first doctor—Smart Patients are way ahead of the game much of the time).

It doesn't matter if this hospital is across the country or, in some cases, in another part of the world, since many specialists can consult from afar. (Some health care organizations even offer an online second-opinion program using their best specialists—check the hospital you wish to use.) The process of finding a superstar doctor for a second opinion is similar to finding a superstar surgeon, so flip back to chapter 3 for pointers. At minimum, find a doctor who's more experienced in your problem than your first physician. There's little point in going to a lesser specialist, obviously.

Stay objective. When a Smart Patient consults a doctor for a second opinion, she gives it the Joe Friday treatment: hands over the test results, gives the facts of her case, and lets us ask the questions. She doesn't say, "My doctor said I have this, but I have my doubts." That's because she knows physicians are human; if your doctor is extremely respected in the field, and we know you're hoping that we'll find a different diagnosis than he did, that could unconsciously affect the way we look at the test results. Instead of just giving our neutral and independent

World-renowned Expert

opinion on the data, we'll almost have to examine the clues and rationale an esteemed professional used to come to a specific conclusion, and that's not quite the same. You don't want your first doctor's work to be checked, you want another physician to approach your case completely fresh, without any preconceived notions.

Smart Patients never bash their first doctor or the testing procedures when getting second opinions, nor do they brag about him and how they're sure he's correct. (The latter can happen when patients are getting a second opinion only to satisfy an insurance requirement). They just give the facts and have an honest, objective conversation about those facts. In short, they avoid saying or doing anything that could bias our interpretation of their history, condition, or test results. This doesn't mean they cloak everything in secrecy; they just don't make it known that they came to us with the specific intent or hope of getting a specific answer.

Your second job? Organize all of your information. We've mentioned your health care advocate—the trusted friend or family member who acts as your partner—several times now. But in case we've been too subtle, getting a second opinion is one process in which your advocate can really play a critical role and take a lot of the load off your shoulders. You're going to be wading through reams of documents, and it'll be very easy to be confused. Your advocate can, as always, take notes and record conversations, and help you sort everything out. You'll need help to:

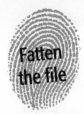

Ask your second-opinion doctor what specific information he'll need. Happily, you probably won't need to retake the same battery of tests you went through to get the first diagnosis; the second doctor may be able to interpret the results you already have. He should give you a basic exam, though, and you'll need to tell him your health history and other important points.

After visiting the second doctor, you'll soon have the second opinion. The final step is to decide what action you're going to take now that you have it.

That action depends on the news you get, of course. In most cases, your second opinion will confirm the first diagnosis. That doesn't mean it was an unnecessary step; this allows both you and your doctor to forge ahead with clear minds. This is a great way to educate your physicians and is often the best way for doctors to learn from one another.

But what if the second doctor doesn't agree with the first one?

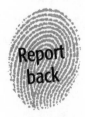

After giving your second-opinion doctor the same checklist of questions you gave your first doctor (see the checklist "By George, He Thinks I've Got It" on page 227), take the info and any new test results back to your first doctor and ask him to review it with you. This is a big test for your doctor; in the very small chance that he acts insulted or indignant at being contradicted, you may need to find another doctor. More likely, you'll have a meaty discussion about the discrepancies in opinions.

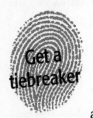

It's sometimes necessary to get a third opinion when the first two disagree, and many insurance plans will pay for it. You won't just be going with the best two of three, by the way. In adding a third diagnosis, there are ways of digesting all of the information to make the most informed decision possible; it's highly likely that your first two physicians both made correct observations, even though they disagreed, and this may mean that you need to take a completely new path than what you had been contemplating.

Boning Up

Just like smart detectives working a case, Smart Patients have saved their own lives (and the lives of relatives and friends) by doing their own research legwork. And having the research savvy of a Smart Patient is never more valuable than in a situation that calls for a second opinion.

The Net Pay

The Internet—it's the nation's daily source of emails, advertisements, international banking scams, weather reports, book and CD purchases, cheap plane tickets, time-wasting jokes, gossip blogs, and so on. Somehow we lived without it until just a few years ago. But how? Surely we were miserable and unfulfilled.

Aside from the uses mentioned above, the vast majority of Smart Patients find most of their health information on the Internet. The resources and access available on the Web are, to put it mildly, staggeringly awesome. You can now learn as much about any condition in fifteen minutes—whether it's diverticulitis or diabetes or insomnia—as it would have taken you three days of library research to learn just a couple of decades ago. What's more, the Internet makes it easy for you to quickly hook up with other human beings who can give you new information and new options for treatment. For better or worse, of course.

Yes, you know all Web sites are not created equal. And much of the medical and health information online is completely wrong, outdated, needlessly frightening, engineered to sell a product or con people, or some combination. Besides using your common sense, and the instincts of a smart detective interviewing sketchy informants, what clues can you use to separate the good sites from the bad ones?

Glad you asked.

While our own field of geekdom doesn't coincide with the field mastered by computer geeks, we've learned how to shake essential and reliable information out of the World Wide Web, and our Smart Patients have taught us much of what we know. For starters, when you're appraising the reliability of any Web site, look at the three letters after the "dot," or period.

A ".com" site is a commercial site. It could be completely legit, or it could be operated by some freak in his basement who's trying to sell you something or con you out of your bank-account number.

The domain ".edu" indicates the site of an educational institution. It is likely very reliable, though the info may not be up-to-date or thorough.

A Web address with ".gov" at the end indicates a United States government site (such as **www.cdc.gov** for the Centers for Disease Control), which is about as trustworthy and fallible as .edu.

There are .org sites, which are usually not-for-profit entities with a relatively high caliber of information. Always check the legitimacy of .gov, .org, and .edu sites; scam artists know that people trust these sites a little more, so many set up fake Web sites using these familiar ending letters for nefarious purposes.

If there is no indication on the site as to its author(s) or the qualifications of the author(s), be skeptical about its content. Before you believe anything you read online, always ask these questions:

How recent is the information? If you see that the site hasn't been updated in months (or years!), the content may be out of date. Don't rely on any medical info that's more than two years old, or on any content found on undated pages that carry an offer to buy discount Enron stock.

Does the Web site contain advertising? Or is it underwritten by another company? For example, drug companies offer Web sites that provide information about prescription drugs they sell, but they may not be unbiased in terms of the data they share or which facts they emphasize (or don't emphasize—think of a politician's speech here). If the company is selling a prescription antacid drug, you can bet that its article about natural acid-reflux cures will determine that all of the natural treatments, in the end, just don't measure up.

Does the site identify the source of the health information it includes? Do any claimed medical facts and figures have references, like the name, date, and journal number of the medical journal it came from? Does it offer links to other non-biased sites, such as government health sites, to confirm this information or learn more about the topic? If the site gives no sources at all or only identifies the information's source as a doctor known as "Freddy," don't trust it. (Sorry, Freddy, but your hair-growth tonic didn't work.)

Does it suggest one specific treatment plan? That's a warning sign.

The Medical Study: Solid, Shaky, or Sham?

"Studies have found . . ."

"An independent study proved . . ."

"Research shows . . ."

"Roizen and Oz are brilliant . . ."

You see these phrases every day. We've used these testaments many times in this book. (Okay, we made up one of them). A clinical study is often the best marker of reliable information in medicine, since it washes out opinion, psychological factors, and other meddlesome pollutants of medical advice. But when is a study trustworthy, and when is it just a lot of air? Before a smart detective would consider a study to be admissible evidence, he'd find out the following:

How was the research conducted? Was it an actual clinical study with live subjects, or a survey, or simply a review article summarizing the published research? Even a straightforward study can be misleading. For example, research shows that people who eat more servings of fruits and vegetables tend to have lower rates of cancer than those who eat less. But while fruits and vegetables are beneficial, this study shouldn't be touted as meaning that they can prevent or cure cancer.

How large was the study? In general, sort of like toga parties, the larger the study, the better. A study of 3,000 people is more reliable than one composed of ten people. How long was it? A study that tracks people for the seven years they spent in college is certainly different than one that tracks them for five days on a road trip. And you probably wouldn't want to do a general study on marriage by interviewing only couples who have been married for three months or less. Right?

Did anyone go blind? In general, you should trust only *controlled, randomized, double-blind* studies. These three research-nerd words simply mean that the subjects were put into groups in a random fashion that wouldn't skew the results. What's more, the researchers themselves were unaware of which subjects were actually being tested and which were in the "control" group. In a drug study, for example, they would be given a placebo—the so-called sugar pill that offers no benefits at all—or another treatment.

Where was the research conducted? A big clinic or university hospital with a solid reputation, or was it in done in a basement in Queens, New York? While we'd never say that you should trust only studies done in the United States, we will tell you that not all foreign research institutions adhere to the same standards of objectivity that our domestic studies do. This is why the FDA insists on seeing some U.S. studies for almost every drug it approves even though the agency will take foreign research into strong consideration.

Who footed the bill? To quote a bit of wisdom we first heard during Watergate, follow the money. If the financial sponsor of the study had a stake in the results, whether it's a drug company or a food company or any private individual, the study is suspect. For example, if a bottled-water manufacturer paid for an expensive study on the difference between spring water and tap water, we wouldn't bet a month's salary that plain old tap water would come out on top.

Miracle Cure or Snake Oil?

Hucksters abound in the health-information and health-product industry, as every Smart Patient knows. It's bad enough when scam artists just sell people bogus products for

hair loss, cold cures, or sexual dysfunction, but it gets much worse than that.
Many unscrupulous marketers target
people with chronic health conditions
and life-threatening diseases, relying
on the fact that they may be willing to
try just about anything in their search
for treatment. Tragically, sometimes
these are the people from whom patients seek second opinions. It
makes us mad, especially when we

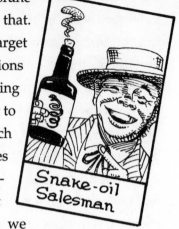

Snake-oil
Salesman

see an infomercial piping a bogus cure right into our own
bedrooms.

You know the adage about something that sounds too
good to be true. Watch for claims supported by unidentified
studies or testimonials from people using phrases like "it
saved my life, improved my sexual performance, and buttered
my bread, too." Be especially wary of testimonials coming
from people who had completely different problems; if a
single product cured one person's dandruff and boosted
another's short-term memory, you can bet it'll do neither for
you. Also be skeptical of products from foreign manufacturers, who may use impure ingredients.

Here are resources you can use to check out health products:

☞ The U.S. FDA's Center for Food Safety and Applied Nutrition
   monitors safety, product information (including labeling and

claims), and warnings and safety information about foods and supplements. Its Web site, at **www.cfsan.fda.gov/~dms/ supplmnt.html,** includes information about supplements.

☛ The FDA offers info about buying medication and medical products online at **www.fda.gov/oc/buyonline.**

☛ To report a health product that you think is being falsely advertised, call the Federal Trade Commission (FTC) at 877-382-4357 (TDD: 866-653-4261), or mail your complaint to Consumer Response Center, Federal Trade Commission, 600 Pennsylvania Avenue NW, Washington, DC 20580. Alternatively, go to **www.ftc.gov** and click on "File a Complaint."

☛ If you think you've been harmed by a supplement or a treatment, report it to the FDA MedWatch by calling 800-332-1088, or file a complaint online at **www.fda.gov/ medwatch/report/hcp.htm.** Your name will be kept confidential.

The Experiment of a Lifetime

There are thousands of medical studies going on at this very minute, not including your youngest daughter's efforts to determine the effects of nonstop boy-band music on hamsters. New drugs, new treatments, and then new follow-up information on old drugs and treatments—the variety is limitless and the supply of info, never ending. The closest you may have ever come to a clinical study is seeing an advertisement in your local newspaper or city magazine that reads, DO YOU

HAVE INSOMNIA? GET FREE DRUGS BY VOLUNTEERING TO BE STUDIED! But there are many more opportunities than that. Whether you're undergoing laser vision correction or open-heart surgery or shopping for an arthritis pain medication or insulin, there is likely a clinical study being conducted that's relevant to you.

The advantage of participating in a study is that you may get access to a new and improved treatment, which can be a lifesaver in some cases. You'll also be en-sured of receiving very meticulous care. There may also be a big cost savings. The downside? The drug or treatment being tested on you might flunk, or you might be in the group receiving the placebo (the fake drug or treat-ment). There's still the warm and fuzzy feeling of donating the services of your body to science while you're still breathing, however. You're helping doctors develop new and better treatments and likely even helping to save lives. You can search through an up-to-date database of ongoing and upcoming medical studies look-ing for volunteers at **www.clinicaltrials.gov**. Another resource is the Thomsom Centerwatch Clinical Trials Listing Service, which is online at **www.centerwatch.com** and lists more than 41,000 studies (you can contact them by phone at 617-856-5900). If you want to participate in a study about an alterna-tive medicine, which we'll cover in chapter 9, click on **www .nccam.nih.gov/clinicaltrials**.

GOOD GOOGLE, BAD GOOGLE

It's a rare sign of success—or at least popularity—when people start using your name as a verb, and it keeps trademark lawyers well employed.

Did you Xerox that file? Did you FedEx it to her? Did you Roizen the nuts and Oz the eggplant?

Well, forget all that.

Just Google this for me, will ya?

Google is one of the newest members of the elite Name-to-Verb Club, as it's claimed its place as the best and most popular search engine on the Internet. But Smart Patients use it only very selectively and very diligently when searching for health information. That's because Google has some big drawbacks when you're looking for objective, correct, and up-to-date info.

Mainly, when you do a search on Google, the results won't just include the good, reliable stuff, it'll bring you everything—all the garbage, all the commercial huckster sites, all the fear-mongering sites, all the old and outdated pages, everything—and nothing will be vetted for quality or accuracy. You'll have to sort through all 290,000 sites to get to the 15 that you really need. Sure, when you know what you're looking for, and it's proving elusive, Google can be golden. Personally, we might use Google—er, we might Google baseball scores—but for health info we tend to cut right to the verified and trusted sources such as many of the sites listed beginning on page 250, and also many of the other Web sites we've recommended throughout this book.

Be Far-Sited

The list below includes some of the best health-research Web sites available on the Internet. A Smart Patient will proceed through the sea of clues like a smart (underwater) detective: be discerning, skeptical, and methodical. And hold any research you find up to the standards we've outlined in this chapter.

Agency for Healthcare Research and Quality

www.ahrq.gov/consumer

This Web site, while aimed primarily at health care professionals, has some health information for consumers as well.

American Medical Association

www.ama-assn.org

The American Medical Association's Web site includes stories about medical issues and news and lets you search for doctors by name or medical specialty.

CDC Health Topics A to Z

www.cdc.gov/ncidod/diseases

This section of the Centers for Disease Control site includes information about infectious diseases, which the CDC studies.

Center for Drug Evaluation and Research

www.fda.gov/cder/drug

This site, part of the FDA's Center for Drug Evaluation and Research, includes information about prescription and over-the-counter drugs, drug safety, and links to major drug-information pages.

Cochrane Collaboration
www.cochrane.org
This not-for-profit organization maintains a searchable database of key clinical studies for hundreds of conditions.

Combined Health Information Database (CHID)
www.chid.nih.gov
The Combined Health Information Database is a bibliographic database produced by U.S. health-related agencies. The database includes titles, abstracts, and availability information for health information and health education resources with simple and detailed search options.

Diabetes Physician Recognition Program (DPRP)
www.ncqa.org/dprp
This site was developed by the National Committee for Quality Assurance (NCQA) and the American Diabetes Association (ADA) to recognize physicians who demonstrate high-quality care to patients with diabetes.

Division of Over-the-Counter Drug Products
www.fda.gov/cder/Offices/OTC/default.htm
This site, part of the FDA's Center for Drug Evaluation and Research, has information about over-the-counter drugs and their safe use.

Drugs.com

www.drugs.com

This site includes a database with drug information drawn from three leading medical-information suppliers; it provides a free drug-information service for both prescription and OTC drugs.

Family Doctor

www.familydoctor.org

This site, sponsored by the American Association of Family Physicians, includes more than two hundred clinically reviewed articles on health topics for men, women, and children. You can also search for physicians who are members of AAFP by zip code.

FDA Kids' Page

www.fda.gov/oc/opacom/kids

This site, sponsored by the U.S. FDA, is designed to help children learn more about drug and food safety.

The Health Library at Stanford Streaming Video Collection

www.med.stanford.edu/healthlibrary/resources/videos.html

This site, a service of Stanford Hospital and Clinics, includes a variety of health-related lectures, classes, and other presentations available online through audio and video.

Health Privacy Project

www.healthprivacy.org

This Web site, part of a nonprofit group, helps raise public awareness about health privacy; it contains information about how to keep your medical records private.

HealthWeb

www.healthweb.org

HealthWeb is a collaborative project of a group of health-sciences libraries and provides hundreds of health, disease, and reference links.

Heart/Stroke Recognition Program (HSRP)

www.ncqa.org/hsrp

This site, developed by NCQA and the American Heart Association/American Stroke Association (AHA/ASA), recognizes physicians who demonstrate high-quality care to patients who have had a stroke or have cardiac conditions.

Institute for Safe Medication Practices

www.ismp.org/consumers/default.asp

This site, managed by a nonprofit organization, provides information to consumers to help reduce the risk of medication errors.

KidsHealth

www.kidshealth.org

Sponsored by the Nemours Foundation's Center for Children's Health Media, this site lets parents, teens, and children learn about hundreds of topics relating to children's health.

National Cancer Institute (NCI)

www.cancer.gov

The National Cancer Institute Web site includes information on many types of cancer and related topics, including treatment, prevention, and coping with the disease; it also includes information about ongoing clinical trials.

National Guideline Clearinghouse (NGC)
www.guideline.gov
This site, created by the Agency for Healthcare Research and Quality (part of the U.S. Department of Health and Human Services), provides treatment recommendations based on the latest scientific evidence for a variety of health conditions.

National Institute on Aging (NIA)
www.nia.nih.gov
The NIA offers information on applying for clinical trials, as well as a wealth of other health resources.

National Library of Medicine (NLM)
www.nlm.nih.gov
You'll find links to sites, resources, and databases that you can use to research health conditions and diseases.

National Women's Health Information Center
www.4women.gov
The site, sponsored by the U.S. Department of Health and Human Services, includes health information specifically for women. It also discusses other topics as well, including minority health, and has dozens of articles in Spanish.

New York Online Access to Health (NOAH)
www.noah-health.org/em/pharmacy/index.html
This site was developed by four New York library associations to provide accessible health information to the public. It caters to the

Spanish-speaking community and includes an index of health topics and resources.

NIH Health Information
www.health.nih.gov
Created and managed by the National Institutes of Health, this site includes information about hundreds of health subjects, with special sections on children's health, minority health, men's health, women's health, and senior health.

Office for Civil Rights—HIPAA
www.hhs.gov/ocr/hipaa
This is the Web site for the federal Office for Civil Rights (OCR), which is responsible for receiving and investigating claims of Health Insurance Portability and Accountability Act violations; includes information about your rights under the law and ways to keep your medical records private.

Patient Advocate Foundation
www.patientadvocate.org
This Web site is sponsored by the Patient Advocate Foundation, a nonprofit group that works to help patients resolve insurance, job retention, and debt problems that result from health problems.

Rand Corporation
www.rand.org
This fifty-year-old research organization conducts surveys and studies on many health issues, often at the policy level, but you can find good info on topics such as HIV, mental health, and insurance.

RealAge.com

www.realage.com

You can take dozens of research-based diagnostic tests, quizzes, and questionnaires on this for-profit consumer-health Web site, and also find physician-reviewed information on common maladies such as back pain, heartburn, and arthritis.

Safe Medication

www.safemedication.com

This site, sponsored by the American Society of Health System Pharmacists, includes information for consumers about using medication safely and appropriately.

UpToDate.com

www.uptodate.com

Find information on medical topics written by medical specialists. This site is primarily for doctors, and a full subscription costs $495 a year, but you can access the "For Patients" information free.

USDA/FDA Foodborne Illness Education Information Center

www.nal.usda.gov/fnic/foodborne/

This site, sponsored by the U.S. Department of Agriculture (USDA) and the Food and Drug Administration, includes information about food-borne illnesses, how to prevent them, and other resources.

8

Just What Gives You the Right?

You Have Rights, You Know. Here's How to Use Them

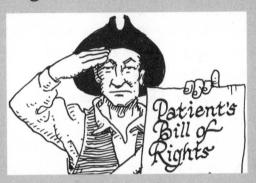

Detectives who've had a run-in with their neighborhood hospital may have noticed one way that suspected criminals are treated better than patients: you can't get thrown in the pokey without learning your rights. Yet you can spend days or weeks in a hospital without anyone talking to you clearly about your basic guaranteed entitlements and privileges. Sure, these things are mentioned in various places in the armload of forms you're given when you're admitted, but are you in the right state of mind to read them when you've just been admitted to the hospital? Most of us just skim these papers, at best. That's not good; if there's ever a time when you really need all the protection that you're entitled to, it's when you're embroiled in the thick of the medical system.

Many of us don't ask about our patient rights when we're undergoing medical care because we probably assume that ensuring our rights is someone else's job. Also, many of us enjoy so many rights in the U.S.A., we often don't appreciate them until something unusual happens (like spending an afternoon trying to ring the American consulate from a Mexican jail—long story).

Seriously, if you tried to tally all of the legally enforceable rights you possess at this very moment, it would probably take you three days. Aside from being inalienably entitled to speak your mind, purchase weaponry, and be tried by your peers on matters concerning sums greater than $20, you enjoy a long list of government-sanctioned rights with nearly every little thing you do. This include buying shoes on your credit card, hopping a cab in Vegas, and—one that's close to our hearts—calling your doctor with a question about your laboratory test results or your upcoming surgery.

Yes, there's a Patient's Bill of Rights. It was created by the American Hospital Association in 1973 and revised in 1992 (see "In Civics and in Health" on the opposite page). The Joint Commission has a long laundry list of your patient rights that it requires its accredited hospitals to honor. Other health care associations have chimed in with their own lists in the years since, as have many individual hospitals. The gist is pretty

straightforward: you are guaranteed
speedy care, full disclosure of costs,
confidentiality, and a bevy of other
civilized basic rights, many of which
you also enjoy when buying a new
muffler for your car. If you wouldn't
be intimidated to ask about your warranty on the muffler, you shouldn't be embarrassed to ask about the warranty on
your knee replacement or your new heart
valve.

Taking the tips we've given you in the
previous chapters will ensure that you
wring the greatest benefits from your patient rights. Many are simply guarantee-
ing your prerogative to do (or not do) the things we've
recommended. However, there are a few extremely important
rights that don't fall into this category, and it's up to you to
take advantage of them. We'll give these rights special attention in this chapter.

In Civics and in Health

The Advisory Commission on Consumer Protection and
Quality in the Health Care Industry (we're assuming this is
one of the shorter names suggested when President Clinton
appointed the group in 1997) created a "Consumer Bill of
Rights and Responsibilities." The Joint Commission also en-

sures that health care organizations respect your rights when providing care, treatment, or services to you or your family. Here are just a few of the basic entitlements you enjoy as a patient in our fair land:

- As a patient, you have the right to considerate, respectful care. You aren't obligated to be considerate and respectful to those who are caring for you, but it would be nice.
- You have the right to obtain current, understandable, relevant information about your diagnosis, treatment, and prognosis from health care providers. Rather than waiting for it to be handed to you, though, we'd suggest exercising your right to seek it out on your own, if you want to add *objective* and *complete* to the adjectives above.
- If you speak another language, have a disability, or don't understand something, you have the right to have it explained to you so you do understand it. This doesn't mean that doctors have to give you the answer that'll make you happy, however.
- You have the right to immediate emergency screening and stabilization when you're in severe pain or have been injured. Of course, immediate could mean sixteen hours if the ER is really backed up that night.
- Except in emergencies where you must be treated right away, you have the right to discuss your treatment options, the benefits and risks involved, the length of recuperation, and medical alternatives before making a decision about your care. You even have the right to discuss this with so many doctors,

consultants, and alternative-medicine practitioners that you might never get around to making any decisions.

☛ You have the right to know the identity of the people involved in caring for you as well as their experience, such as if they're new residents or students. You can attempt to flirt with them as well, but it may not get you better treatment.

☛ You have the right to know the estimated costs of all treatments. You also have the right to be given ice water and a cold compress after fainting upon learning the estimated costs.

☛ You have the right to make decisions about the care you'll receive and to refuse certain treatments to the extent permitted by law. In the best situation, you won't have angry relatives trying to have you declared insane.

☛ You have the right to expect that your medical information will be kept confidential, except in cases where reporting it is required by law. For an example of the latter, if you have the Ebola virus, we have to report it. But you won't have too long to be upset anyway.

☛ You have the right to have an advance directive such as a living will, durable power of attorney for health care, or health care proxy. This is one of the main reasons we wrote this chapter, in fact. (Don't get confused by all the terms; an advance health care directive is a document used in some states that combines a living will and health care power of attorney.)

☛ You have the right to review your medical records and have the information in them explained to you. You may also express consternation if your medicals are presented to you in seven large supermarket paper bags, and you're given a pitchfork to sort through them.

☛ In a hospital setting, you have the right to receive medical care within a reasonable time. Reasonable is a much longer span of time than immediate, and immediate is subject to the interpretation explained in a previous right.

☛ You have the right to agree or refuse to participate in research studies and to have them fully explained to you before you jump in. This doesn't guarantee that a treatment will be named after you, however.

Is This on the Record?

Some of the most significant (and controversial) rights you enjoy as a patient concern the information included in your medical records. Even if you're not a celebrity, your overall health record—if assembled in one place—would likely be fatter than the congressional tax-code book. It's stuffed full of reports, microfilms, and other media with a similar topic: you. Each time you visit a physician or enter the hospital, more information goes into that file. Eventually all the info will be stored on computer CDs, but eventually could take a long time.

ID Thief

You're probably just envisioning laboratory test results,

physician notes, maybe copies of bills, and the like. But your medical record contains much more than that—much more—and this is why it can be tapped by your insurance company or another organization in case of a lawsuit or other legal issue. You might think of it as a credit report for your body. (Let's hope it's one that would clear you to qualify for at least a fifteen-year mortgage.) What's in that file? Among many other things, you'll find:

☞ Consent forms. You've signed dozens of these in your life; perhaps hundreds, if you want to count elementary-school field trips. Naturally, you'll have to sign one before undergoing any surgery or medical procedure. These often have little value, since most folks would not bother coming to the hospital for a procedure that they don't want if they were conscious when they came, that is), but the devil is in the details. So pay attention to those details and read the consent form carefully to make sure that your name is spelled correctly, the described procedure and site of your surgery are correct, and the like.

☞ Consultations. These are usually a fancy name for second opinions, which we discussed in chapter 7. Any reports made by doctors other than your primary physician (such as a specialist) get thrown into the consultation category.

☞ Discharge summary. If you've been hospitalized, your records will include everything noted about your stay, including your diagnosis, test results, and procedures and their results, as well as your condition when you left the hospital. Doctors sometimes use poetic license to cram a two-week hospital stay into one paragraph, so a Smart Patient will read the discharge summaries (or ask someone to translate all the gobbledygook) before it's tossed into his health file for posterity. If that condensing caused some important events from your hospital stay to be missed, you have a right to correct that.

☛ Medical history and physical information. This is all the basic stuff that you neatly consolidated for **Your Health Journal** in chapter 1, such as any illnesses and surgeries you've had, any current medical conditions and medications you're taking, your family history, and so forth. This part of your file will also include your doctor's notes from appointments, which might make for entertaining reading. Doctors aren't supposed to gossip in these sacred notes, but things tend to fly out of our pens during examinations. You can take a trip down memory lane and revisit any or all of your illnesses and maladies by going through these notes, if that kind of thing turns you on.

☛ Immunization history and record. These records will show which shots you received and when, which will save you time and trouble if you step on a rusty nail and need to quickly find out if your tetanus protection is up-to-date. When you book that dream vacation to Mozambique, you'll be able to see how many needlesticks you need to increase the odds that you'll return as happy as when you left.

☛ Pathology reports. If you had tissue removed and analyzed during surgery, the analysis of the tissue (was it cancer or not?) will be here, written up in all of its undecipherable subcutaneous glory. Hopefully all these analyses will correspond to specimens that you *wanted* removed.

☛ Physician's orders. These are the specific directions your doctors gave you after specific appointments and procedures. Don't worry, the file won't say whether you followed the orders—unless that was all too obvious to your doctor during a subsequent visit.

☛ X-rays and imaging reports. While X-rays, mammograms, and ultrasound films and visual records are usually kept in the radiology department or on a computer, your medical record will usually include the written findings describing those images. More recently, however, digital images are being stored on computer disks and in your doctor's or hospital's computer system, so accessing them (with your permission) is easy for second-opinion docs and others.

Now, in the ideal situation, all of this information will be in your medical record, neatly tabulated and logged, legible, and current. The odds of that being the case, of course, rival the odds that you'll have your own CBS sitcom next year. Health workers called health information management professionals are responsible for keeping your records complete and accurate, but that's an extremely difficult task, given how mobile most people are. Your medical record is likely scattered among several different physicians and a few different hospitals, if you're like most patients. However, like your credit report, the medical record maintained for you by your last few health care providers or insurance companies you've dealt with probably contains a large chunk of comprehensive info, even if it's not a perfect and complete dossier. The increasing use of computerized records is one reason for this.

What does this have to do with your patient rights?

Most of us are concerned about having someone peek into our private lives for unscrupulous purposes, whether it's an employer, a life-insurance firm, or our future in-laws. Obviously, whoever has access to your health record—with or without your permission—can learn more about you than you probably remember about yourself.

Let's Keep This Between Us

Confidentiality. It's one of the hottest topics in health care today. Imagine all the ways that troublesome medical info could be used against us, especially in this blessed computer age of immediate worldwide data sharing (which saves many lives every day, of course). The classic questions abound: What would happen if your employer accessed your medical record and found out that you had HIV? What if you're running for town council, and someone tries to find out if you've ever received mental-health treatment? Could a new insurance company refuse to cover you if it found out you successfully underwent cancer therapy seven years ago?

The people who offer cut-and-dried answers to these questions are usually doomsday prophets or uninformed about the complexities of these thorny situations. The health care industry isn't ignoring the issue of security, however. We know you care about keeping your medical records secure from prying eyes as much as you care about having curtains on your bedroom windows (or even more, if you're like our neighbors), so huge efforts are being made to protect this information.

One of the biggest steps to protect privacy came in April 2003, when Congress passed the Health Insurance Portability and Accountability Act (HIPAA). It was sort of a stepson of the Freedom of Information Act for you; and, on the downside, a bit of a Lockdown of Information Act for us. This act still didn't reveal who shot JFK, but it did make you and your doctor sign many more forms (what government law doesn't increase cost and paperwork?). And it guarantees you the right to see your records. HIPAA allows you to look at, request changes to, and get copies of any health-information documents kept about you and your care. When it was passed, physicians had to send a letter to every single patient, asking them to sign consent forms; surely you remember having your mailbox stuffed with these odd, out-of-the-blue letters back in the spring and summer of 2003, don't you? Well, in case you didn't read those missives too closely, we'll summarize them for you. Specifically, HIPAA gives you the right to:

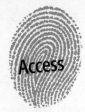

Access

You can see, supplement, and copy your health records. If you want to review your medical records, request them by contacting the doctor's office or hospital where you were treated. Usually you'll sign a release-of-information form; it may ask you to specify the information you want. You may also be asked to pay a reasonable fee, such as 10¢ a page, for copies of the records. Hey, nothing's free anymore.

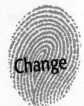

Change

You can request that your medical records be amended if they're incorrect. You can do this by contacting the health professional who made the entry (such as your doctor) or the health information management staff member at a larger medical office or hospital. If your request is denied, you can have your written request put in your file.

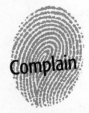

Complain

If your privacy has been violated, you can file a complaint with the person at your doctor's office, hospital, or insurance company who's responsible for handling privacy issues. If that doesn't give you satisfaction, you can formally complain to the Department of Health and Human Services' Office for Civil Rights by calling 800-368-1019 or going to **www.hhs.gov/ocr/hipaa**.

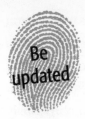

Your doctors, hospitals, and insurance companies are required to inform you about their privacy practices. You'll probably receive the notice on your first visit.

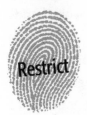

You can request that the use and disclosure of your health information be restricted to certain purposes. Your doctor or hospital doesn't have to agree to your request, however, and may still be legally forced to share your info in certain circumstances (in case, say, you have a communicable disease or one that's recorded in state records). To be honest, the privacies mandated by HIPAA weren't exactly an earth-shattering revelation. Staying mum on private matters has always been part of our profession, as it is with lawyers, bartenders, and hairstylists. According to the American Medical Association's code of medical ethics, your doctor has a duty to maintain the confidentiality of everything you two discuss, so you can feel assured that everything you tell your doctor stays with him or her. If you don't get that vibe, talk it over or find another doctor. Of course, if you casually mention that you're going to drive your car off the lip of the Grand Canyon, he or she might have to breach that confidentiality to stop you from harming federally protected land.

Your state may have laws that are stricter than HIPAA, by the way. To find out, contact your state's department of health or click on Health Privacy Project's Web site, at **www.health privacy.org.** Also, you can further guard your medical info with a couple of commonsense moves, such as not giving your name or other info to Web sites that don't guarantee privacy (unless you're currently receiving too little junk mail, telemarketer phone calls, and sexual-enhancement spam, that is). And don't blink into autopilot and obliviously sign the next seemingly routine consent form someone hands you at work, or the doctor's office, or elsewhere. Learn who specifically you're agreeing to give access to your info and why. (Really, does the local cable company need to know when you had your last colonoscopy?) Finally, let your doctor know any specific worries you have about the privacy of your records.

When HIPAA Hurts

As with every seemingly necessary law, such as the ones about paying income tax and not "borrowing" other people's cars, HIPAA brings some inconveniences along with all of the good it does. Chiefly, it makes it difficult for your doctor and other parties to share or access your medical information, even in emergencies. That's mostly a good thing, but most Smart Patients want their doctors and specialists working together as easily as possible, especially in an emergency. Making sure that your doctor can share your info with another physician on a moment's notice can be a much more important concern—since it could save your life—than worrying about broken confidentiality. A Smart Patient, like a smart detective, works best when all of the team members are in sync and have the same info at their fingertips. Giving your doctor permission to share your information is an important Smart Patient move; you don't want to get wrapped up in red tape when you're already covered in bandages.

Also, you can avoid a lot of hassles in trying to get information from one physician to another by making sure that you have all of the info in your hands first. That way, you can personally give it to the new doctor or a lab without bugging an intermediary who's constrained by privacy laws, such as your primary physician or the original lab. To make this easier, every time you go to the doctor or see a specialist or get a test done, ask for a copy of your record from that day's visit right then and there. It'll cut down on later phone calls and faxes and aggravation trying to dig up data after the fact. So before you leave, always get a receipt of what you had done that day. And just like at a fast-food restaurant, remind them that all services are free if you don't get a receipt. Don't push for the smile, though.

YOU'RE A CARD

It seems now that everyone has one of those little "thumb drive" storage devices for their computers, the kind that are about as big as a lipstick tube (or, um, your thumb) and can hold thousands of pages of data. You can slip it into your pocket or carry it on your key chain and then stick it into your computer and bring up the amount of info you once needed six hundred computer diskettes—or a dozen large cardboard boxes—to stow. Maybe we've been reading too much science fiction, but, really, how long can it be before each of us is carrying our whole health file in our pocket, along with our DNA sequence and every phone book in the world? And how long before we inadvertently give it to a parking lot attendant?

The U.S. Department of Health and Human Services beat us to this thought. If the folks there have their way, soon you'll carry your entire health record in a container that's so thin you could use it to jimmy open a door. They've been busily creating the futuristic-sounding National Health Information Network (NHIN), which will make the health records of each and every (willing) American accessible on the Internet and may allow us to carry copies of our digitized records in something resembling a credit card. With one swipe or download from your key chain and a password from you (was it the dog's name or Aunt Mable's street address?), a new doctor will have all of your health info immediately.

A specialist in Oregon will be able to call up your X-ray online and discuss it with your primary-care doctor in Georgia, who's looking at the same digital picture. There will be no waiting for test results to be sent from the lab to your doctor and then to

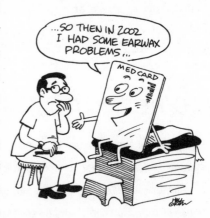

...SO THEN IN 2002 I HAD SOME EARWAX PROBLEMS...

MED CARD

another physician. Drug prescriptions might be checked against the online records, to prevent dangerous errors and potentially save thousands of lives every year.

Of course, there are some things that still need to be worked out, such as how the network will function, where the data will be stored, how records will be protected, what laws will govern its use, and other such trifles. While this network sounds like an Orwellian nightmare to some people, a survey found that 72 percent of Americans like the idea—just so long as the privacy protections are rock solid. Given that major credit-card companies still have their databases hacked fairly frequently, that second part may not be the easiest feat. We especially don't want your boss peeking into your file; 68 percent of survey respondents want the data off-limits to employers.

We'd say stay tuned, but you'll probably have time to tune out and tune back in long before this is ready for a test drive.

Rights That Matter Right Now

A living will. Health care power-of-attorney form. Do-not-resuscitate order (or DNR, in health lingo).

Who says paperwork is the most boring part of medicine? Opting out of important contracts like these has authored some of the most exciting (and controversial) moments in health care in the last twenty years! Relatively few people take advantage of these patient rights, so there is still plenty of day-to-day action to be seen. The court cases, the relatives throwing chairs, the television cameras—who needs Jerry Springer? As long as you and other Americans overlook these measures, by thinking they're just too grim, too unlikely to matter, or just too complicated to figure out, there will be no end of these thrilling scenes to enliven our workplace.

Now, if you don't want to become a participant in these dramas, you may want to look into your patient rights and complete some of these contracts. We'll go into each just in case.

Living Will

Those two words evoked about as much emotion as "life insurance" did not long ago. But that was before Terri Schiavo captured the country's attention in 2005. You probably remember her story. It was in all the headlines for quite a while. Terri was only forty-one, but she lived in what several doctors believed was an unresponsive "vegetative state" with no hope of recovery after experiencing heart failure fifteen years before. Her husband maintained that Terri had once told him that she wouldn't want to live under such circumstances, and he took legal measures to have her feeding tube removed, which would have eventually brought about her death. Schiavo's parents objected, saying that she wasn't unresponsive, could recover, and had never expressed the wishes that her husband claimed. In any event, she had left no written instructions. The hospital removed and reinserted her feeding tube twice, while legal battles ensued. In the end, the law sided with the husband.

Had Schiavo made a living will—not something that

many twenty-six-year-olds do, admittedly—the whole messy affair may have been avoided. The media exposure had hundreds of thousands of people gasping, "That could be me!" and living wills became a vogue subject, even among people younger than forty. Simply, a living will is a document that explains which medical treatments you want and don't want if you have a life-threatening illness or are too sick to voice your own wishes. A pre-Schiavo survey found that only 20 percent of Americans actually had a living will, although that figure is likely higher now, and it's at least double that among Americans older than seventy.

You don't need a lawyer to write a living will, although talking to one about it isn't a bad idea. As a Smart Patient, you will also talk this over with your doctor, too, since you want to make sure your directions are as informed as possible. State laws differ about when living wills can be used, and your lawyer (or your hospital) will know the specific rules. Remember that a living will is consulted only when you can't speak for yourself. Some patients get anxious by wrongly thinking they might be giving the hospital or a relative a free ticket to bump them off in case they annoy them. But that won't happen. Unless you specifically want it to, of course.

The forms for living wills are easy to fill out. (At least, once you've made the hard decisions about what you'd like done in case you're incapacitated.) They vary among states, but you'll find a common example in appendix 2. You should give copies to your health care advocate, family members, doctors, lawyer, trusted friends, and maybe also your dog if he's proven to be more reliable than other members of your household.

Aside from unexpected catastrophes, a living will can make a big difference in the comfort and control a person experiences as he's getting closer to, well, negotiating the final sales transaction of his private agricultural acreage. Researchers have found that people with living wills receive better treatments to keep them comfortable and pain free as they near the end of their lives, as compared with patients without living wills. They are also more likely to die in their own homes or in a nursing home instead of in a hospital, in case that appeals to you.

Health Care Power of Attorney

While a living will tells people what you'd like done in several nonpeachy circumstances, a health care power of attorney form (also called a durable power of attorney for health care or a medical power of attorney) designates a specific person to make decisions for you, which is a handy thing to have for a couple of reasons. First, something may crop up that your living will didn't predict. Second, you won't have six relatives battling over who should be in charge if you can't talk for yourself (and risk having the nephew you never liked prevail).

The person you deputize as your decision maker may be the same person as your health care advocate (your partner in all things medical, first explained in chapter 3 on page 102). Or it can be your spouse. While current spouses are the legal next of kin and almost always have power of attorney, this doesn't mean a family member (or even the U.S. Senate, as Terri Schiavo's husband found) won't contest their decisions. But having a formal health care power of attorney document makes their wishes a firmer extension of your own.

The person you designate to call the shots for you, either for a finite one-time treatment period or in perpetuity, might be called your agent, attorney-in-fact, proxy, or surrogate. Who should it be? You should have someone in mind now, since thousands of people a day, unfortunately, end up needing health care proxies in a sudden, unexpected manner. To have peace of mind, a Smart Patient would put it in writing when he or she is well. You should also talk this issue over with your parents and/or children, and, if applicable, any other relatives who may not have a clear health care proxy available. Again, if you leave this issue to be hashed out when it's an emergency, there's a good chance that your family meetings will be free theater for everyone in the hospital.

Obviously, being a proxy is one heck of a responsibility, and this person must be up to the task—mentally, physically, and emotionally. Your proxy needs to be comfortable with the role (well, as comfortable as possible), and confident that she or he can do the job. And your proxy needs to be someone you can trust, because this is going to take teamwork. So choose a partner you can count on to stick by you when the going gets rough (think Starsky and Hutch). The three qualities you need your proxy to have, aside from those that prompted you to have absolute trust in this person in the first place, are:

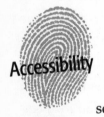

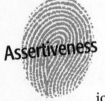

Assertiveness A proxy must be able to state your wishes and stay firm to them amid differing opinions from relatives and hospital staffs, yet still be open minded and discerning enough to know if some bit of exceptional new information warrants a possible change in plans.

Starsky & Hutch

Accessibility If the person lives in Moscow (and you don't), or it takes nine phone calls and four reschedules from personal assistants to see her, she's not going to make a good proxy. You need someone who can be available quickly and give you her attention for undetermined periods.

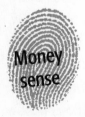

Money sense There's a good chance that the person you pick to be your health care proxy will also be your financial proxy (having it be the same person can ease things considerably), so this person has to know how to handle a buck—and be able to understand and follow your instructions on how your finances should be allocated for your care.

If there's no one in your circle you'd trust to do this or who wouldn't faint at the mere mention of it, don't feel bad; you're not the first one to be in that pickle. Don't feel compelled to just pick someone; a bad choice can be worse than no choice at all. Consider tapping a professional. Some hospitals have staff members who can serve as patient agents, such as social workers and chaplains, although state laws allowing this vary. Some will do this gratis; others charge a fee. Your attorney can give you more options on hiring a proxy. Your doctor usually can't be your proxy, unfortunately. It's a conflict; if he goes against your wishes, he'd have to sue himself. Even if you don't name a proxy, you should still have a living will. If the wording you use in the living will makes it utterly clear exactly what you want, and your living will is known to hospital staffers who treat you (and you need to make sure that *both* are the case), your wishes will be followed.

A way to hedge your bet? Name a backup proxy in case the first one is unwilling or unable to serve just like the first runner-up in the Miss America Pageant—though nude photos will not get your proxy off the hook quite so easily.

What if you have seven children and five siblings, and they all (1) want to be your health care proxy and (2) are qualified to be your health care proxy? This is actually a big problem for some people (with numbers slightly fewer than seven, though), since not appointing a person to be your health care proxy is a bit like not inviting a friend or relative to your wedding; it's a tangible act that can be viewed as drawing a line in the sand between who really counts for what, no matter how logically or nicely or gently the decision is made. There's no easy answer here, except to deputize the person you feel most comfortable with and to name number two the backup. Then tell everyone else, saying that you love them too much to put them through such grief and burden. Letting them fight it out to decide who can be your proxy? Nah. This is your choice, so don't leave your proxy vulnerable to being second-guessed by everyone who cares about you. That's why the Constitution spells out a line of succession for president; otherwise the original document could have simply allowed us to pick whoever's especially smart and available at the moment.

Speaking of original documents, a sample durable power of attorney form is in appendix 2, your doctor or hospital can give you forms specific to your state. State laws vary, so make sure that the form you're using complies with your state's requirements. Note that some states require that a witness also sign the document, so flubbing that will make it invalid.

Do-Not-Resuscitate Orders

You can opt for a do-not-resuscitate (DNR) order even if you don't (yet) have a living will or health care power of attorney. Straightforwardly, this means that if your heart stops or you stop breathing, the medical staff won't try to revive you. You have to specifically ask for a DNR and put it in writing (as in the sample form from Illinois in appendix 2), two measures that most people find reassuring. If you don't ask for a DNR order, you'll get the default "RLC order" (resuscitate like crazy).

It could pay to ask the hospital staffers how you would be marked if you elected DNR status. A bizarre occurrence a few years ago highlights this. You may recall seeing the yellow rubber wristbands that some people wore to show their support for cancer patients. You know, the ones from the Lance Armstrong Foundation? Well, patients began showing up in hospitals wearing these wristbands, which unfortunately look exactly like the ones some hospitals give patients who don't want to be resuscitated. This caused alarm and confusion, but luckily nobody was sent to the hereafter due to a screw up. The best part? The rubber wristlets from the Lance Armstrong Foundation are called "Live Strong" bands. That's the peak of irony or the perfect motto of a do-not-resuscitate philosophy.

On Second Thought...

Except for the sphinx, nothing's carved in stone, right? Sometimes we change our minds. Or other people change our

THE LIVING TRIO

In your living will, you can tell hospital staffers ahead of time—if things should take a particularly unhappy course, and you can't speak up for yourself—which measures you do or do not want to receive, such as:

ARTIFICIAL BREATHING

No, not via the personal services of one of the more attractive hospital staff members, we're afraid. A machine called a ventilator pumps air into and out of your lungs.

ARTIFICIAL FEEDING

If you're unable to eat, you can be given nutrients through an IV or a tube that's inserted into your stomach. Some of our more industrious friends have asked if they could have this procedure done just as a matter of convenience, but we tell them they work too hard as it is.

CARDIOPULMONARY RESUSCITATION (CPR)

The organized theatrics you've seen in countless TV shows and movies, when a hospital team tries to revive you after your heart stops beating or you stop breathing (unless you request a do-not-resuscitate order, that is). Unlike on television, however, there is not a 99.9 percent chance that you will be revived successfully and to full consciousness within five seconds by a tanned actor, but we'll try our best.

minds. If you've completed a living will and health care power of attorney and then decide that you want to make changes, it's not difficult. Just tell your doctor, your designated proxy, and all other relevant parties, and update the documents. Make sure you destroy all of the old copies and replace them with new ones; you don't want multiple versions floating around. Before making changes, however, you may want to sleep on it. It's easy to get angry at the kids for doing something irritating and to suddenly think, "I *do* want to be a burden to them," but the delayed satisfaction may not be worth the administrative hassles.

Checklist: Broach in Case of Emergency

In Chapter 7 we reviewed the questions you should ask your doctor when you've been given a diagnosis. But what if it's that kind of diagnosis—the kind in which you not only want a second opinion but also need to think about some of the disturbing issues we're dealing with in this chapter, such as living wills and health care proxies? This Smart Patient checklist will give you all the information you need to mobilize a health care team to fight a serious illness and to make some tough decisions that could bring peace later on:

☐ How is this illness likely to affect me? What kind of effect will it have on my family?

☐ What kind of decisions may I have to make as my illness progresses? What can I do to prepare for those decisions?

☐ What kinds of symptoms am I likely to experience in the future?

☐ What are the best and worst outcomes I can hope for or prepare for as I face this illness? Remember to ask about experimental and in-development treatments; the answer to this question could change tomorrow.

☐ If my disease is terminal, what is the longest and shortest amount of time I can expect to continue to live? Take either answer with a grain (or a wheelbarrow) of salt, by the way. A study of doctors' predictions has shown that we are often off, sometimes by years. Sometimes by decades.

☐ Will you promise to speak openly and honestly with me, and others whom I choose, about my illness, prognosis, and treatment alternatives?

- [ ] If I become unable to participate in my care or speak for myself, how will decisions be made for my care?
- [ ] If I designate a proxy, are there any specific decisions my proxy should be prepared to make in dealing with this illness?
- [ ] Will you help my family and me locate resources such as spiritual support, social workers, or hospice care, if I need them?
- [ ] If I choose hospice care in the future, will you continue to care for me?
- [ ] If I am in a nursing home, assisted-living facility, or at home, will you or someone you recommend make house calls to see me?
- [ ] What can I do now to help prepare to fight or manage my disease? What resources can you suggest that I explore?
- [ ] If an emergency arises, who should we call?
- [ ] If I decide that I do not want to be resuscitated, how can I ensure that my wishes are carried out?

Are the Organs Stayin' or Goin'?

Your clear orders for your immediate postlife adventures should include your wishes on an autopsy; if there's no mandatory medical reason to perform an autopsy, do you still want to have one done? In deciding this, weigh two things with your other considerations. First, your children will be able to use the autopsy information to better gauge their own genetic health risks, as we mentioned in chapter 1. Second, if your doctors or the hospital staff made a medical error or misdiagnosed you, your autopsy could reveal their mistake, as we mentioned in chapter 7. Sure, that info could be quickly shuttled to a team of rabid attorneys, but bringing the error to light might also save the next patient who's at risk of falling victim to the same mistake.

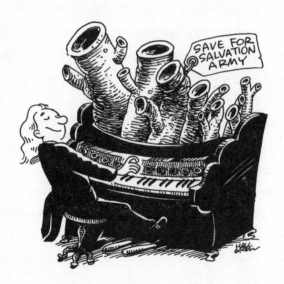

Also, do you (or a loved one for whom you might speak one day) want to donate organs to needy recipients or be a specimen for needy med-school students? Why, that's wonderfully generous. Just put it in writing, please. You can state this intention a thousand times, and everyone may know you've intended to donate your organs since you were a wee child of ten, but if even one of your relatives objects at the last minute, it likely won't happen unless there's written permission from you. Don't give your evil nephew the satisfaction of yanking away one of your last magnanimous acts.

You Are the Proxy

The only thing that's potentially harder than facing your own life-threatening illness is helping a family member or a close friend engaged in that battle and being the person entrusted to make sure the patient's wishes are followed. If you are called to perform this duty for an aging parent or your husband or wife, it can be emotionally wrenching, since you're dealing with your own grief, sadness, and fear while trying to be strong and responsible. But you may also feel fortunate that you're there to help. We can assure you that this will almost always be one of the most poignant journeys of your and your loved one's lives.

The information you need depends on how large a role you will play as that person's proxy, whether you are an immediate relative, and how much control is granted to you. Asking the following questions will help you determine where you stand. They'll also give you specific ideas on what you'll need to talk over with other family members, the person's doctor, hospital social workers, and an attorney.

☛ What's the person's diagnosis and prognosis?

☛ How certain is the answer to the above question? What are the odds of a partial or full recovery? Because predictions are often wrong, you don't want family members to start vying for possessions prematurely.

☛ Has the person prepared and signed advance directives? If the person has not, and he or she is able to, for Pete's sake, try to get it done! This could save you tons of stress and hassle.

☛ Has the person spoken with any close friends or relatives about what his or her wishes would be in the event of an incapacitating injury? Hopefully you'll be the one spoken to, but if not, better to find this out now rather than later.

☛ Does the hospital have a social worker, ethics committee, or other staff members to help you consider the available options for care?

☛ What kinds of financial assets does the person have? No, you're not snooping (well, that shouldn't be your motivation); you need to know this in case you have to answer questions about what type of care he can afford and his eligibility for programs like Medicaid.

☛ Does the person have medical, long-term care, or Medicare insurance that will cover the cost of hospital or long-term-illness care? It's always a happy occasion when he does. (If you don't, you can read the preceding sentence as a recommendation to look into long-term-care insurance and other provisions, so you'll cause a happy occasion if that question comes up in your case one day.)

Please Stay In-formed

In appendix 2, Sample Forms, you'll find examples of a living will, durable health care power of attorney, and do-not-resuscitate order. Since these particular copies are from the Illinois Department of Public Health Web site and there's a fair chance that you're not in Illinois at this moment, remember that they're here only as references. So please don't rip them out and use them, though we encourage that with almost everything else in this book. You can get these forms from your doctor or your hospital.

9

Considering the Alternatives

On Pins and Needles About Acupuncture and Herbs? Here's What You Need to Know About Alternative Medicine

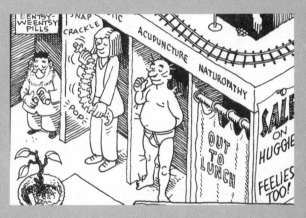

Fifty billion dollars. No, it's not the cost of a Humvee according to Pentagon accountants, but that's a good guess. It's what Americans spend on alternative medicine treatments every year. Running the gamut from drugstore vitamins to chiropractors, acupuncturists to herbal remedies, massage to hypnosis, the country is crazy for complementary and alternative medicine (CAM). They're termed "complementary and alternative" because they're usually meant to complement traditional medicine, and—although many seemingly could be more mainstream or common—they're outside the fray of conventional medicine.

There's good reason for the zeal that many people have for some CAM treatments. A few of the therapies have been around for millennia and have strong track records of success, and some have proven their effectiveness in clinical studies. As physicians, we're happy to have these disciplines in the healing arena and to work with their practitioners because we see many patients benefit greatly on a daily basis.

Do you sense a *but* coming? You know us too well by now.

Of course, while a large number of CAM professionals have their patients' best interests in mind, shams abound. There are plenty of hucksters peddling unproven rip-offs, designed to rid patients of their cash rather than their health complaints. Some are dangerous, too. The deaths caused by weight-loss supplements that contained large amounts of the stimulant ephedra are a vivid recent example, but thousands of other people are saddled with problems every year because of abuse or impurity in this unregulated, hype-ridden industry. Don't be too gullible or believe everything you're told is based on proven studies. You can't bumble your way through the world of alternative medicine as if you were Inspector Clouseau and expect to stay out of harm's way.

Okay, you can see we've got our skeptical hats on, but, again, we must emphasize that we're not against alternative medicine at all. We're just bothered that patients think the alternative part means it's an alternative to *us*: we boringly conventional, science-minded, Western-schooled doctors. We make it our business to know as much as possible about these treatments and use them whenever we think they'll be safe and helpful. And they can be particularly helpful if you have a chronic problem that requires ongoing treatment or when our fine conventional medicine is, shall we say, stumped. Even the mystical end of CAM isn't off the table for us. Hey, if detectives use psychic profilers on dead-end cases and occasionally

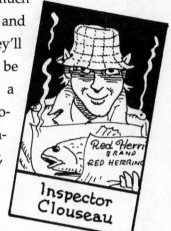

get to the perp's front door, our minds are open to trying alternative medicines. You might even find us shopping at Green Gene's Alternative Mall (see the next page).

Let Us in on Your Little Secret

We know from research that about three out of four patients are using some form of alternative medicine right now, whether it's nightly prayer or gulping what they believe is the herb yohimbe in hopes of better bedroom sessions. But how many patients tell us that they're using alternative medicines? Fewer than one in five. That rankles us, because (1) we're in the healing business and detest being kept in the dark in case you've

À la Mode Alternatives

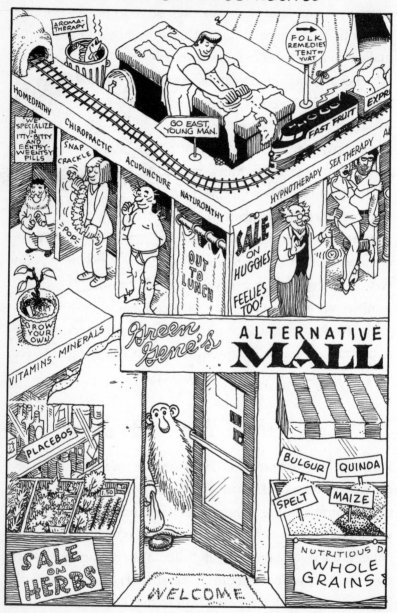

found a great thing, and (2) we could send you home with a prescription that could inadvertently send you to the morgue.

So tell your doctor!

Sure, you may not feel that it's critical to call us on a Saturday and say, "Doc, I forgot to mention that I say five Hail Mary's every night" (though we'd actually appreciate knowing that for academic sake, since prayer is being clinically studied). We're chiefly concerned with anything you swallow, inject, absorb, or undergo that has a physical component to it, obviously. But we understand your reluctance to tell us; most patients think their physicians just scoff at an alternative treatment, even if we don't know a thing about it. Those patients are sometimes right, if they're seeing one of the more rigid doctors with a dusty diploma.

Just What Are We Talking About?

How would you best define alternative medicine?

a. Something that is less expensive than "real" medicine (like, um, surgery)

b. Something that complements conventional medicine (like cranberry sauce on turkey)

c. A substitute for conventional medical care

d. Things that haven't been shown scientifically and are not valid enough to be mainstream

e. Anything or anyone someone can sell for cash that will supposedly fix something that's wrong with you

When a Gallup poll put this question (more or less) to the deans of medical schools, most chose *d*. In other words, they say that if there's no science, the treatment is not conventional. What about when there *is* science? Why, then it's no longer alternative, in their definition. The therapy can be called mainstream, and this has happened with such treatments as taking aspirin to reduce heart-attack risk, or meditating to fight hypertension.

Although conventional doctors think alternative medicines haven't gotten the scientific stamp of validity, alternative practitioners bristle at the implication that their therapies aren't as effective as clinically proved medicine. There's truth in both sides. No therapy was born proven, and clinical studies cost truckloads of money and often won't be done unless someone can recoup that cash with sales—and no one has the exclusive patent right to sell, say, cod liver oil. This means that you have to decide which alternative therapies you want to explore and ultimately have faith in. Many that have at least been proved safe—at least to the extent possible—don't have a firm, scientific verdict on their effectiveness. You're the one-person clinical study when you take it, and, as we like to say in America, your results may vary.

Show Us Proof—Pretty Please

While many practitioners of alternative therapies were once able to work without licensing or proof of formal training, at least by U.S. standards, that's no longer the case for many of them. As doctors and Smart Patients discovered that specific alternative treatments were highly effective (tugging them closer to the mainstream-medicine category), medical groups created credentialing standards for them. However, the Joint Commission doesn't accredit alternative medicine practitioners yet.

We'll go through the most common complementary and alternative medicine fields below—the ones you're likely to encounter in a strip mall or city office. We'll start with those that have the most rigorous standards and work down to those that, well, are the most friendly to people looking to start second careers.

Now, even though this list is ranked in order from the most regulated to the least, we're not passing judgment (lest we be judged, with hate mail and rotten eggs, most likely). Just because a therapy appears lower on our list doesn't mean that it can't be safe and beneficial in the hands of a skilled practitioner. And just because it's higher up doesn't mean it's been proved to work or deliver on all of its claims. Also, keep in mind that requirements vary from state to state, so the health commissioner's office in your state should be able to tell you the credentialing standards for specific alternative medicines and therapies.

Let's Talk Back: *Chiropractic*

We all ache back there, and millions of us use a chiropractor to ease the pain, help our posture, or achieve other health benefits. Chiropractors are licensed in all fifty states. Back whackers, as some skeptics call them, must study for four to five years (or get 4,200 hours of training) at one of sixteen accredited chiropractic colleges recognized by the U.S. Department of Education. They also need to pass a four-part exam. Unlike conventional doctors, however, DCs don't need to do an internship or residency. Some states and insurance policies

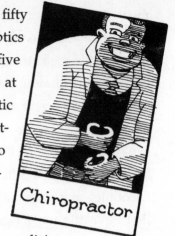

Chiropractor

give chiropractors more powers (such as to be someone's primary-care doc) than others do. The Federation of Chiropractic Licensing Boards Web site **(www.fclb.org)** is a good info source. Research has found that chiropractic treatment is just as effective in getting most back patients back to their normal routines as the treatments offered by conventional physicians.

Stick 'Em Up: *Acupuncture*

The ancient Asian therapy of placing tiny needles into specific areas of the body for countless purposes—from stemming chronic pain to smoking—is one of the most popular CAMs in the United States, and also one of the most regulated. Thousands of physicians practice acupuncture, and they need no additional licensing in any state. Acupuncturists without a medical degree require licensing in all but eight states, which entails training and passing an exam. Some states also require a hands-on exam. About sixteen states require a degree from a school accredited by the Accreditation Commission for Acupuncture and Oriental Medicine (ACAOM) and the other twenty-six states require three years or 1,800 hours of training. In about twelve states, your doctor must refer you to the services of an acupuncturist before insurance will consider paying for it. To find out what your state requires, check the National Certification Commission for Acupuncture and Oriental Medicine (NCCAOM) Web site at **www.nccaom.org.**

Doing What Comes Naturally: *Naturopathy*

Naturopathic doctors (NDs) don't use drugs or advocate major surgery; they opt for healing agents that come straight from the earth, or at it, such as water, air, and sunbeams. Most states have no credentialing requirements in naturopathy; only eleven require licensing, and there are only four naturopathic colleges, all accredited by the Council on Naturopathic Medical Education (CNME). The naturopathic doctor curriculum is a four-year postgraduate program with the first two years covering natural sciences and the second two covering clinical sciences. There is a national exam on basic sciences, laboratory medicine, nutrition, minor surgery, and several other areas. You can find your state's status at the American Association of Naturopathic Physicians (AANP) Web site, **www.naturopathic.org.**

Full disclosure: Many conventional doctors aren't too keen on naturopaths calling themselves doctors, because some feel that this could confuse patients and cause them to think that they've had the same training. Smart Patients know the difference between MDs and NDs, and DOs and DCs, and even DC3s and DC10s at the airport.

What Doesn't Kill You Makes You Stronger, Right?: *Homeopathy*

Homeopaths believe that giving an extremely tiny dose of a substance that can cause sickness allows the body to safely build defenses against the real disease. Only three states (Arizona, Connecticut, and Nevada) offer homeopathic licensing for physicians, but there are about 6,000 practitioners of homeopathy in the U.S. Most are practitioners in another field, such as chiropractic, naturopathy, veterinary medicine, or physical therapy. If you live in one of the forty-seven other states, find an MD or DO who is board certified by the American Board of Homeotherapeutics. Note that in Arizona and Nevada, homeopathic assistants can practice under the supervision of a homeopathic MD or DO. For info, see the North American Society of Homeopaths Web site at **www.homeopathy.org.**

Research on the effectiveness of homeopathic medicine has not been conclusive, and one large study recently published in the *Lancet* medical journal found that it offered no greater benefits than placebo (or fake) treatments in most cases. Homeopathic docs disagreed with these findings, of course.

It's Rub-bish: *Massage*

Credentialing requirements vary more for massage than for any other alternative therapy. Half of U.S. states require a minimum of about 500 hours of in-class (a must for our masseuses, personally) and supervised training at an institution accredited by the Commission on Massage Therapy Accreditation (COMTA). Only 42 of the approximately 1,000 massage schools in the United States have this accreditation, by the way. Therapists must also pass various exams. Some states require continuing education varying from three to twelve hours per year, too.

Other differences also exist. For example, some states distinguish between a "registered" massage therapist, who has 500 hours of training, and a "certified" massage therapist, who has an additional 60 hours of college credits and is permitted to practice in a wider range of settings. Also, there are states where regulation is done at the level of the town or city. The other half of U.S. states have no credentialing requirements at all, although there's a lot of infighting about this. Check out the rubbers in your state at the National Certification Board for Therapeutic Massage and Bodywork (NCBTMB) Web site, **www.ncbtmb.com.**

The Hyp Cats: *Hypnosis*

Hypnotherapy is the least regulated of all CAMs. Forty-eight states have essentially no licensing or training requirements at all, which makes us wonder if hypnotists don't visit their governor every now and then with their swinging pocket watches. Only Illinois and Oregon are trying to implement licensing requirements.

Hypnotherapists can buy very official-sounding licenses from official-sounding organizations, most of which look impressive on their business cards but don't mean a whole lot otherwise. The irony? Hypnosis has been in the United States longer than any other CAM, and it can be one of the most effective complementary therapies when combined with conventional health care. We've seen benefits from hypnotherapy done by licensed psychiatrists, clinical psychologists, and skilled social workers. There have been plenty of studies with varying results, and the National Institutes of Health is currently conducting clinical trials to see if hypnotherapy can reduce surgical pain and tension, hot flashes in breast cancer survivors, and other ailments. If you'd like to explore being part of a study, go to **nccam.nih.gov/clinicaltrials/hypnosis .htm.**

For more info and referrals, see the Web site for the National Guild of Hypnotists, **www.ngh.net,** which is a fifty-year-old nonprofit organization with a good reputation, as well as the American Psychotherapy and Medical Hypnosis Association Web site at **www.apmha.com.**

Checklist: Find Your CAM Man (or Woman)

You want to find a reputable alternative-therapy practitioner and not get soaked or scammed? Take these steps.

☐ **Ask your doctor if he or she will collaborate** with an alternative-therapy provider, and ask for referrals.

☐ Dial the insurance company. Some CAMs are covered, and others are for your wallet to bear alone. Likewise with different CAM practitioners. **Find out your insurer's specifics.**

☐ Ruthlessly **check credentials.** Find out how many years the CAM provider has been practicing, and call your state's professional, licensing, or occupational regulation offices to see if he's properly licensed or has any nasty happenstances in his history. For unlicensed fields, such as aromatherapy and biofeedback, you'll have to rely on a trustworthy referral and your gut instincts.

☐ Make sure the CAM practitioner is **open to conventional medicine** and will work with your doctor's therapy (and doesn't insist on being the alternative to your doctor's therapy). If he scoffs at conventional medicine, we'd run out of there. But that's us.

☐ **Research the therapy** before you visit the practitioner. Scam CAM providers love uninformed patients. Two great sources are the National Center for Complementary and Alternative Medicine Web site at **www.nccam.nih.gov**, and the National Library of Medicine's Directory of Information Resources Online at **dirline.nlm.nih .gov**; the latter allows you to search a database of thousands of alternative-medicine organizations.

☐ **Find out when you can stop the therapy.** "Never!" is a bad answer. That can mean the practitioner is hoping you'll not only be her patient, but an ATM. Some ailments will require ongoing treatment, but check the validity of the claim with your doctor.

The Supplement Story

The biggest connection most people have with alternative medicine isn't hypnosis, massage, acupuncture, or anything they do to their bodies, it's the herbs and nutritional supplements they put *into* their bodies. A simple multivitamin and herbs like ginkgo biloba—they're examples of edible alternative medicine that millions of Americans have no trouble swallowing every single day of their lives.

Is that good or bad?

Our honest answer: yes.

Like space, the ocean floor, and all issues theological, what we know about the benefits and harms of nutritional supplements is dwarfed by what we don't know. And to quote a recent secretary of defense, we don't even know what we don't know.

With the exception of a few basic vitamins (C, D, E, B_5, B_6, B_{12}, folate, niacin, and A) and a few minerals (calcium, magnesium, selenium, potassium, and iron), we have limited scientific information about most of the supplements on the market. One of the most frustrating aspects about the millions of pills lining drugstore and health-food-store shelves isn't that they don't work, but rather that we don't have proof they actually *do* work.

Sure, for many minerals and vitamins, we know the minimum amounts of essential nutrients needed for survival—the recommended daily allowances (RDAs) or the daily values (DVs). But we know very little about the optimal doses you should take of those minerals and vitamins to prevent, slow, or even reverse diseases and age-related maladies. We'd love to say that the claims you hear from health-food-store employees and infomercial hosts are all unqualified bunk or that much of it was right on target, but we just don't know yet. There have been few or no

Natural Foods Store Clerk

large, controlled scientific studies on the majority of nutritional supplements, so their effectiveness (and even safety) is part faith and part conjecture. Because there's little hard evidence, marketers can claim anything or nothing at all, both of which can greatly mislead buyers. Most supplements are sold without any description of what they are, why they are supposedly good for us, or how we should take them. It still boggles our minds that this is legal.

Soft Claims Versus Hard Drugs

What's the difference between the drugstore herbal supplement and the prescription medication sitting side-by-side on your nightstand? They're about as different as a pound mutt and a pedigreed dog. Before a company can sell a prescription drug, it must be subjected to several meticulous, costly clinical studies. Manufacturers have to compile a mountain of data showing that the drug is safe and does what it claims it does. The company then has to submit all these data to the Food and Drug Administration for approval—and that can be a notoriously difficult feat. If all of this effort comes together, and the company can afford the millions of dollars it takes to complete this process, the drug will one day debut in a pharmacy near you.

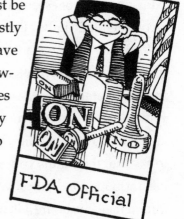

FDA Official

After that, the company continues to conduct quality checks. It will test the pills to make sure that the millionth one to roll off its conveyor belt has exactly the same potency as the first lonely little orb that dribbled off the factory line. Even with all of this meticulous testing, there's still a fair chance that the drug will cause unforeseen problems when taken by thousands of people.

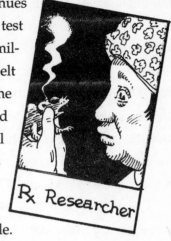

Rx Researcher

In comparison, all any pill manufacturer—or a single ambitious person—needs to do to sell a nutritional supplement is, well, sell it. It can be a motley concoction that contains almost any substance, and the seller needn't prove a thing.

Impure Thoughts

Why is this the case? Nutritional supplements are classified as food products, not medicines, so they aren't regulated by the strict standards governing the sale of prescription and over-the-counter drugs. Manufacturers can sell them in any quantity or combination they want, and as for quality control, let's just say it's *eclectic*. Different brands of the same supplement might contain wildly different ingredients. They'll frequently contain contaminants not listed on the label. Buy two bottles of an herb such as saw palmetto from two manufacturers, and they may each contain a substance different from the other—and two that bear no resemblance to saw palmetto. Yes, the law allows this!

Since 1994, the Dietary Supplement Health and Education Act (DSHEA) has permitted herbal remedies to be sold in the United States as food products. The second paragraph of this law states (and we paraphrase): "What is on the [bottle] label may or may not be in the bottle. And what is in the bottle may or may not be listed on the label."

Can you imagine if aspirin manufacturers were given the same leeway? We could have brands that contain no aspirin whatsoever, and others that pack ten times as much as the label declares. Manufacturers would also be free to market aspirin under the name that Native Americans knew it by, cinchona bark, which would add dozens of interesting possibilities for confusion or deception.

Luckily, there's one easy precaution you can take. Whenever we buy a nutritional supplement, we always look for the "USP-verified" mark on the label. This means that the United States Pharmacopeia, a reliable nonprofit science organization, has tested and verified the supplement. It's the best evidence you'll get confirming that the pills actually contain what the manufacturer claims they do. Check out the U.S. Pharmacopeia's Web site at **www.usp.org** to get more details about the organization.

Given such wide variances in their products, why aren't we seeing hundreds of deaths a day caused by impure nutritional supplements? Most include too few active ingredients in their pills, so you're often taking nothing more than a placebo. The Food and Drug Administration has very little authority to mess with nutritional-supplement companies because they're not drug manufacturers; they're selling foodstuffs or nutraceuticals (natural substances believed to have health benefits), according to some decision made decades ago. Further, the FDA can't even inspect the company's manufacturing process unless it has reasonable evidence that its products are harming people—and this means some people need to be harmed before the FDA can step in. That's a little late, if you ask us.

Vitamins: Do You Need Them?

What do we actually know about vitamins, minerals, and other supplements? Which ones should you take? Which ones should you definitely not take? In general, if you eat a balanced and healthy diet, with four servings of fruits, five servings of vegetables, and plenty of grains, you should get most of the nutrients you need through your food.

However, most of us have busy lives and hectic schedules, which means that it's not always easy to eat a balanced and nutrient-rich diet. In fact, of the more than 15 million people who have reported their diets on the **www.realage.com** Web site, fewer than 80,000—less than 1 percent—get the right amount of vitamins D, B_6, B_{12}, and folate, and the minerals calcium and magnesium, from food alone. Taking a daily multivitamin can help pick up the slack. We'd choose a multivitamin without added iron and one that has less than 2,500 IU of vitamin A and beta-carotene, combined.

If the only time you get close to fruits is when your in-laws visit, you'd be wise to take a multivitamin twice a day; several vitamins dissolve in water, and you urinate them out so your body cannot benefit from them for more than twelve hours. Other good candidates for a two-a-day regimen are calcium (because your body can't absorb more than 600 mg at a time) and vitamin C.

How healthy is your diet? Your doctor or a nutritionist can tell you. Vitamins can be especially important if you're a vegetarian or follow another special or restricted diet. Make sure you're taking in at least 800 micrograms of vitamin B_{12} a day as well as all essential amino acids, because vegetarian diets skimp on these necessities. A tip? Incorporate quinoa into your weekly menu; it's a grain that has all the essential amino acids, and it tastes great.

Ready, Willing, and Herbal

Many Americans swear by herbal medicines, and we believe there's good reason for their enthusiasm. Even though the data aren't rock solid yet, there's no doubt that many herbal supplements can deliver strong benefits. But they also carry dangers, and that's where we get a bit anxious about the fervor over these au naturel treatments.

In fact, we prefer to call herbal supplements by another name. One that's more accurate.

We call them *drugs*.

Several herbs are potent substances that can cause strong effects in the body—desired and not. Even if they don't pose a danger by themselves, herbs can affect the absorption, circulation, metabolism, or excretion of other substances in the body, such as prescription medicines. For example, taking St. John's wort, a popular supplement that some research suggests may alleviate symptoms of depression, can accelerate the metabolism of birth control pills. In other words, taking St. John's wort as a happy pill may lead to a little unexpected bundle of joy. Further, the safety of mixing common herbal supplements together is still a big question, and we see a lot of patients who eat more herbs in a day than your average locust swarm. These patients are graciously volunteering to be guinea pigs in their own informal clinical studies.

Two herbs that patients ask us about more than any others are ginkgo biloba and ginseng. Ginkgo biloba comes from the leaves and seeds of the Chinese ginkgo tree. Many people think it can boost memory, lower blood pressure, and even reverse aging. Ginseng is a root that's taken as an energy booster, and some people also believe it can strengthen the immune system. Do these two hugely popular herbs work? Patients want a definitive answer. So we give them one: Try the supplements, and if they work for you, then, yes, they work.

There are plenty of studies on these herbs, but their results are contradictory. Most of the evidence for them comes from personal testimonials and anecdotes. And, for the reasons we've already mentioned, it's often impossible to know what's really in a bottle of ginkgo biloba or ginseng based on the label. What one supplement manufacturer calls "ginseng" another may call "garbage." Even if the pills genuinely contain these herbs, their potency can vary greatly. It can even depend on the time of year the herbs were harvested. (Again, hunting for the little "USP-verified" mark will help ensure at least some consistency.)

The bottom line for all nutritional supplements with shaky data is the same: if it's safe and it works for you, then we'll consider it effective. Whether you're taking ginkgo biloba or ginseng, or coenzyme Q10, alpha lipoic acid, glucosamine, L-carnitine—the list goes on for hundreds of drugstore-aisle miles—your only real concern is whether the supplement brought about the benefit you were hoping for, whether it lowered LDL cholesterol, raised HDL cholesterol, increased libido, or anything between. That's the ultimate burden of proof a Smart Patient demands, and it doesn't come from a clinical study or an FDA report.

WHAT'S WHITE, CHALKY, AND TASTES LIKE BARK?

Aspirin was once an herbal remedy. Its main ingredient, acetylsalicylic acid, is found in willow bark, which has been used to treat headaches for more than three hundred years. (Who first decided to chew on bark while he or she had a headache, we'll never know.) Ever since the German scientist Hermann Dressler isolated aspirin in its chemical form more than a century ago, our vanities have had one more medicine bottle taking up space.

Aspirin is also the perfect example of the good and bad that come with herbal remedies. It's friendly when used correctly, but downright rabid when abused. Taking half an aspirin daily can reduce your heart-attack risk because it inhibits blood clotting and inflammation, but the same nuance of chemistry that makes aspirin offer this benefit also causes stomach irritation and even bleeding. Taking no more than 162 mg of uncoated aspirin a day, drinking half a glass of warm water before and after swallowing the pill, and taking the pill one to two hours after eating can reduce that risk. It also helps to never confuse aspirin with ibuprofen and acetaminophen—the pain killers in Advil and Tylenol, respectively—because they're completely different drugs. Another marvelous perk of aspirin? New research shows that taking a daily aspirin when you undergo some types of surgery can help you avoid later complications associated with inflammation. These data are new in the last several years, so many physicians may not yet accept this use of aspirin.

Warning: Don't Mix with Surgery

No matter how much you love 'em, you have to quit taking certain supplements for at least a week before surgery and stay away from them for as long afterward as your doctor instructs; otherwise you could turn yourself into an unfortunate statistic. One set of common consumables you should stop taking a week before surgery is the "G family": garlic, ginger, ginkgo biloba, glucosamine, and ginseng. These can seriously increase the odds for bleeding during surgery. Below is a longer list that we give patients, but it's by no means complete; let your surgeon and your anesthesiologist know everything that you take well before you're being wheeled into the operating room, because many of these supplements (and we do mean supplements with high doses of these substances— not the sources from your dining room table) stay in your bloodstream for several days.

Stop taking this supplement a week before surgery . . .	Because . . .
Dehydroepiandrosterone (DHEA)	These supplements can
Eicosapentaenoic acid (EPA)	affect blood clotting after
Fish oils	surgery.
Garlic	
Onion	
Vitamin E	
Feverfew	These can interact with
Ginkgo biloba	warfarin, a common blood-
Coenzyme Q_{10}	thinning drug, and possibly
Ginger	cause bleeding or clotting.
Ginseng	
Glucosamine	

Stop taking this supplement a week before surgery . . .	Because . . .
Hawthorn berry Kyushin Licorice Plantain Uzara root Ginseng	These can interact with digoxin, a heart drug that many patients receive during and after surgery, and the interaction could be fatal.
St. John's wort	St. John's wort can interact dangerously with a number of drugs, including digoxin, warfarin, oral contraceptives, cyclosporine, and antiviral drugs.
Iron	This mineral can reduce the bioavailability of other drugs.
Caffeine	It can affect your blood pressure, and caffeine withdrawal after surgery causes headaches. Ask for a cup in the recovery room if you're a java junkie.

Making a Cold Call

Come cold and flu season, we see hordes of patients taking echinacea to ward off a budding bug. An herbal powder derived from the leaves and stems of the coneflower, echinacea was a popular folk remedy, and some limited research suggests that it can boost the body's natural immunity. Unfortunately, the very few studies on echinacea in Germany and the United States have produced mixed results. Some found an immune-system benefit, but others found no positive effect. And a few even hinted at negative ones. At this stage, we really don't have any proof as to whether it works or not, and the most current research is pointing to the latter. You might be better putting your money toward a piping hot bowl of chicken soup—which has been proved beneficial by scientific research and Grandma.

10

Take Control of Your Health Insurance

It's Your Most Important—and Expensive—Health Resource. Are You Wasting It?

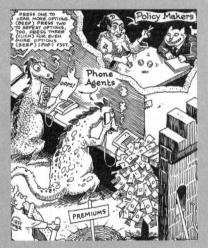

Ask anyone anywhere in the nation about his or her most important problem in health care, and you'll hear one answer almost exclusively. And it's not the high cost of Preparation H.

It's health insurance. As if we have to tell you that.

Before even the Smartest Patient can think about finding the right doctor, or finding the best hospital, or deciding which prescription drug to take—before making any medical move at all—there's one question that we all need to ask. And sometimes we don't like the answer.

What will my health insurance allow me to do?

We'd love to think that you could skip this step, but you can't. For doctors, health insurance is one of the most influential factors we deal with in practicing medicine, just under saving patients' lives. It drives almost every medical decision we make, including which tests and procedures we can use to diagnose and treat patients, and even which patients we care for. Doctors act independently of this concern usually only when making life-and-death decisions, and *usually* is the operative word.

Given the strong influence they exert, insurance companies are an easy target for ire, and everyone loves to take potshots at them. Of course, this isn't fair. Ethical health-insurance companies are using your money to improve the quality of the health care you receive, and they fight to keep costs low—two services that no Smart Patient takes for granted, even if paying the insurance premium is a pain in the neck. In fact, health insurers do a lot of bargaining on your behalf; they routinely use their heft to negotiate discounts of up to 60 percent off hospital service fees and up to 80 percent off

Bean Counter

physician charges for their members. We'll bet you're sending holiday cards to plenty of people who haven't done as much for you. Their reputation as cold-hearted penny-pinchers? In controlling the purse strings of health care, health-insurance companies have to be hardnosed; they must set boundaries and play by the rules, and you would too if given their task. Instead of vilifying health-insurance companies for this, Smart Patients learn these rules so they can use them to their advantage.

You now know how we really feel, so we apologize in advance for all the fun we'll have at the expense of insurance companies in this chapter. We're only human, you know.

G'head, Take Their Pick

Of the 240 million Americans who have health insurance, 60 percent get their coverage through their jobs. Most of the rest have Medicare or Medicaid. If you're among the two-thirds, we'll bet your employer makes it pretty easy for you to make decisions about your health-insurance coverage. You receive your company's benefits-selection form every fall and are given at most three choices in health-insurance plans—which are often variations from the same carrier. Then you read the fine print, and you find out that choices B and C are actually only available to employees in other states. Congratulations! You've just picked insurance plan A. Now, you realize that your human-resources department didn't contract Plan A to be the best choice for *you;* of course; they chose it because it seemed like the best and most cost-effective choice for the largest number of employees.

Given the scant choices, it's easy to see why most people put more thought into ordering at McDonald's than choosing a health-insurance plan.

A Tragedy: Uncovered

Nearly forty-six million Americans (almost 16 percent of our population, including 11 percent of all children) have no health insurance. One reason is lack of availability. Surprisingly, about one-third of U.S. employers (mostly small businesses, the type that built this country and are still chiefly fueling its growth) don't offer health insurance to their workers, often because they can't afford to do so. The high cost of individual policies is another obvious culprit; health insurance ain't cheap, as we all well know. Of course, aside from the people who genuinely can't afford to pay the premiums, there are people who go without insurance and decide to gamble with their financial futures. Why pay $5,400 a year for something they may not need, they figure. Of course they'll need it sooner or later—and you can bet it'll be sooner, most likely at 3:30 A.M. on some fated Tuesday morning when you meet the gambler at the ER and have to wait in line behind him. About 1 in 5 uninsured Americans get most of their care at the local hospital emergency room, and more than 30 percent of those visits are not truly urgent. Yes, they may be quite sick, but they're using the ER for something that could be—or could have been—handled easily at a doctor's office. Given that they receive almost no preventive care, they're also more likely to become ill. Uninsured people are 50 percent more likely to be hospitalized for an avoidable problem than those who have health insurance.

There's help available. People without health insurance should call the insurance board in their state; to date, thirty states offer coverage for low-income residents who are uninsurable. They can also visit the Web site from the Department of Health and Human Services at **www.hrsa.gov/osp/dfcr** and click on "Obtaining Free Care." Two other good Web sites are **www.insurekidsnow.gov** and **www.covertheuninsuredweek .org**. Finally, the Patient Advocate Foundation's site at **www .patientadvocate.org** is run by a nonprofit that helps patients resolve insurance, job, and debt troubles that result from health problems.

If you know someone who's simply avoiding paying for health insurance to save money for a gambling binge, let him know that he's really using that extra cash to gamble with the equivalent of a life-threatening illness. Being uninsured endangers your life more than having diabetes; about 18,000 Americans aged twenty-five to sixty-four die every year as a result of being uninsured, slightly more than the number killed by diabetes.

A Fearsome Foursome

Health insurance is health insurance is health insurance, correct? Please. You know by now that nothing involved with medicine is that simple! Health plans come in more flavors than gelato. But luckily for sanity-loving people everywhere, they can all be sorted into four broad categories. Your health insurance is a version of one of these.

Indemnity Plans

These are the oldest and most liberal plans, the one your dad may have had when he wore the gray flannel suit to his job in 1950. Even up to the 1970s, most Americans still had indemnity plans (also called fee-for-service plans). Your parents (and their employers) paid a lot for this plan, but they may not have complained too much because (1) there was no other choice, and (2) the coverage was wide and largely unrestricted. They could see any doctor, anywhere, and get any medical service they wanted. After paying a deductible (today it may be $500 to $2,000 annually), they would pay a portion (say, 20 percent) for every service they got, from blood tests to baby delivery.

About 1 in 10 Americans with employer-paid health insurance have some version of an indemnity plan. These policies are fairly expensive because the insurers don't require members to use specific hospitals or doctors, so these insurers often get no discount for services. (Insurers who limit their members to "in-network" hospitals and doctors can negotiate huge discounts with those providers because these insurers are guaranteeing them a steady supply of business.) Indemnity plans can be the best choice for people who want ultimate freedom and are willing to pay the higher premiums and co-payments, and don't mind dealing with extra paperwork.

Point-of-Service Plans

Imagine the trusty ape-to-human evolutionary chart, now reverse its direction, and you'll see the (de?) evolution of these plans. The indemnity plan is the fully upright, dignified realization of health insurance. But when indemnity plans began suggesting—but not demanding—that patients use a preselected network of doctors who agreed to give their members discounts on services and supplies, the point-of-service (POS) plan was born. Anthropomorphically, its back is slightly stooped, and its knuckles hang just a tad closer to the ground than the indemnity plan. You still have the choice of using any physician and getting any service, without a referral from any doctor, but you'll pay more (usually a lot more) for using out-of-network docs and hospitals. The premiums usually run a little less than traditional indemnity plans, and there may be less paperwork because your doctor's office will likely have frequent (if not daily) contact with the insurance company.

Health Maintenance Organizations

Ah, HMOs. The most maligned insurance plan on earth, and the one that made us accustomed to the utterance of "managed care." They're way back at the monkey's uncle end of the evolutionary scale. Alas, we're out of order, because things got worse before they got better; insurance had to get this basic and limited before more choices came as a response.

You likely know the drill with HMO plans. They're the least expensive variety because they're generally the most restrictive. Although many different versions exist now, in the traditional HMO you must pick a primary-care doctor who is in the HMO network of physicians, and this doctor coordinates all of your care. That doctor must refer you to specialists who are generally also in the HMO network; you can't just go see them (or any out-of-network doc) on your own whim and expect the services to be covered. You pay next to nothing (or nothing) for in-network care, meaning the care or services you receive from one of the hospitals or doctors who have agreed to accept greatly reduced payments from the HMO's members. But if you see a doctor outside the HMO network, or break the rules, you pay 100 percent of the costs. About a third of all Americans who get their insurance through their employers have HMOs as their health-insurance providers.

Preferred Provider Organizations

An evolutionary step just a sliver closer to proud and noble Indemnity Plan, PPOs were created for people who still wanted economical coverage, but more freedom of choice than HMOs offer. These plans may have a simian crease in their palms, but they are clearly human and a tad more humane. They allow you to use doctors and hospitals outside the PPO network, but at a higher cost. For their mixture of freedom and relative economy, these plans are the most popular in the United States. About 40 percent of people with employer-sponsored health insurance have a PPO plan.

This Is Medicare on Drugs

We all know and love Medicare, which is our federal insurance program that helps Americans who are age sixty-five or older or who are disabled pay for hospital care, doctor visits, and some other medical costs. It's very similar to the health insurance you likely have now, in that you'll pay premiums, deductibles, and copays to use it—though it won't be nearly as expensive as getting private health insurance. (Don't confuse Medicare with Medicaid, which is a supplemental insurance for persons who have very little or no income or savings, and is often used to pay for nursing-home costs.) There was always a big hole in Medicare—namely prescription-drug coverage—which the government attempted to address by adding Medicare part D in 2006. (We're still getting to know part C!)

Medicare part D is a prescription-drug benefit program that helps pay for 146 different types of prescription drugs identified by the U.S. Pharmacopeia (for a definition of this organization, see page 308 in chapter 9). Medicare part D isn't free, it isn't perfect, and it generated a lot of flak nationwide when it was first laid out from people who thought it did far too little to help older Americans pay for incredibly expensive prescription drugs. But it's the plan we have, so let's learn to use it.

The premium for part D is about $35 per month, and enrollees have to pay a $250 deductible before Medicare will cover 75 percent of drug costs until the total reaches $2,250 (and that can be reached in a blink, given the cost of some common medications). After that, you'll have to pay the entire cost of all your prescriptions until you've shelled out another cool $2,850, making the combined total spent on drugs $5,100. After that, Medicare will cover 95 percent of drug costs approved by the plan. Whew! Keep your fingers crossed in hopes that the Washington pack dreams up something simpler and more affordable before too long. Meanwhile, prescription drug cards are one of your best ways to reduce your medication expenses; flip to page 164 in chapter 4 to check them out.

FORGET ABOUT FINDING MY ARM, JUST CALL THE CLAIMS HOTLINE!

Consider them family. If you have a health emergency, your insurance company wants to know about it right away. As in ASAP. Before your mom knows, even. Read the fine print in your policy, and you'll see that, in some circumstances, they can refuse to cover you if you don't call them before you head to the ER or within several hours of arriving. Considering that an ambulance ride can cost just slightly less than a Space Shuttle mission, it's a good tidbit to remember. And, really, what's the trouble? Once you get one finger on your spouting bleeder, just use another one to punch the phone pad. To make it easier, why not put the twenty-four-hour claims hotline on speed dial, right below your favorite pizza joint? In being practical, having your insurance ID number handy will smooth your experience at the ER anyway, and you can be sure that your insurance card will magically vanish from your wallet or purse because it's the first time you've really needed it in the last fifteen years. So the phone call could prevent a common holdup. And your relative or friend can do it for you. (Your advocate, if available, would naturally be the best choice.) Just remember to keep the nice folks down at insurance central in the loop, lest they cut you off like a rambling neighbor.

How Healthy Is Your Health Insurance?

If you actually have a choice among several different health insurers, you either work at a fabulous company (buy stock!) or you have several shiny new cars parked on your property. Even if neither is the case, you'll still likely have a choice between at least two insurance companies, even if it's just between taking your spouse's employer's insurance plan or your own.

This momentous decision can mean the difference between heaven and . . . hassles, if you have a serious health situation. There are thousands of health-insurance companies, and your policy—no matter what you're promised in the contract—is only as good as that company; in other words, a fantastic plan from an irresponsibly run or near-bankrupt insurance company is worth about as much as the Sears Tower deed you bought from that fellow behind the bowling alley. Be a sly detective and find out if the company is shady—or sinking—before you entrust your life and sacred fortune to it. Check its story with this interrogation sheet:

☛ Does your doctor make a troubled face when you mention a specific insurance company? Always, but always, ask your doctor and his or her administrative staff (the billing manager is your best bet) for their opinions on an insurance company you're considering. They get to know these insurers in a very intimate way. Our Smart Patients never hesitate to ask, "My job will be adding a health insurance plan from XYZ Company in the spring. Would you advise me to switch to them or keep the company I have?" Be perceptive; your doc may not want to bash an insurer by saying something as blunt as, "They'll treat you okay, but they continually shortchange me, and I'm going to drop them as soon as I have enough patients from another insurer." The look of acute gastritis on his face will speak volumes, however.

☛ How does the insurer score? Managed-care plans are regulated by federal and state agencies. Indemnity plans are regulated by state-insurance commissions. Phone your state department of health or insurance commission and ask about the insurer's record; ideally, they will not be squealing about any sanctions or bankruptcies.

☛ Have any of their clients hollered fraud? The National Association of Insurance Commissioners (NAIC) Web site (www.naic.org) is a gold mine of insurance info, and most important, you can check out individual companies using its "Consumer Information Source" database. You can also report an insurance scam on the site.

☛ How does the insurer rate with the National Committee on Quality Assurance? Check its Web site at www.ncqa.org. An "excellent" score means its claim handling is superior to other insurers. And speaking of claim handling . . .

☛ How quickly does the company pay claims? This is a big question, because you want that check to arrive in your mailbox before you're too old to drive to the bank. The staff in your doctor's office will give you the scoop. If the company is no good in this category, it's plain no good.

☞ Does the company offer a variety of products and plans? The best insurers will offer at least two plans to clients, even if your employer chooses only one of their plans to offer you. Insurers who offer only one plan are shaky, because they are blocking your ability to customize a program.

☞ If your plan is an HMO, how much cash does the insurance company have on hand? An HMO plan should have 10 percent of the previous year's expenses in reserve. Your state department of insurance or the state insurance commissioner's Web site can reveal if the company's reserve has fallen below its minimum.

☞ Has the insurance company existed for more than five years? Half fail within the first three years, so think twice about going with a new company.

☞ Does the CEO have more than ten years of experience in health care? He or she ought to. Look at the CEO's bio on the insurer's Web site. Several insurance-company CEOs actually have no insurance experience whatsoever. For example, they may have been president of a bank holding company that acquired the insurer in a hostile takeover. Read between the lines; a CEO resume that spouts off a litany of investment firms but shows no direct experience in health care wouldn't make us feel extremely confident if we were shopping for an insurer and had another choice.

☞ If there's a network, how does the insurer choose its doctors? Is there a credentialing process, or are all the physicians board-certified by the American Board of Medical Specialties? For more on board certification, see page 73 in chapter 2. You can verify that the physicians in the network are board certified by checking them out at **www.abms.org.**

☞ By what criteria does the plan choose hospitals? Cost should not be the only factor. Of course, all the hospitals should be Joint Commission–accredited. Ideally, the insurer should also choose its in-network hospitals based on outcomes data, which is the statistical rate of success a hospital achieves in treating certain conditions.

☞ Does the insurer have many doctors clustered in a small geographic area, with a narrow mix of specialties? Ideally, you want to see at least a few doctors within comfortable driving distance (unless you have a private chopper, of course), with at least the major specialties represented. This should include anesthesiology; cardiology; critical care; ear, nose and throat; gastroenterology; general surgery; neurology; oncology; orthopedics; rheumatology; pediatrics; pulmonology; and the specialty you care about if it's not listed here. If the plan has lots of doctors, but they all subspecialize in rare tropical infections and share an office complex that's 272 miles down the interstate, keep hunting.

☞ What is the appeals process? Learn what you'll need to do to fight a claim denial. How many hoops will the insurer make you jump through? (Or, apt to the illustration on page 333, how many moats with alligators will you need to swim across?) The staffers in your doctor's office can give you the lowdown on this too. Above all, make sure that you'll be able to eventually make your plea to a doctor on their staff, and find out at what point that would happen. See "You Will Not Be Denied" on page 337.

☛ What is the insurer's appellate process for doctors? If your doctor will have great difficulty being removed or added to the roster, that could be bad for you. As in any marriage or partnership, if your doctor is unhappy, you will eventually become unhappy too.

☛ What kinds of treatments are considered experimental? If the rest of humanity is eligible for the life-saving albeit expensive procedure, you might deserve a shot as well. After all, that's why they call it insurance. Generally, government approval is the litmus test. That means the FDA and the CMS (Centers for Medicare and Medicaid Services) have agreed that the procedure is worthy. But seeing if other major insurers in your area are covering a procedure is an excellent means to test the waters of eligibility, because our government agencies often take years to formally evaluate a new procedure. Surprised?

☛ Does the insurer survey its members on their health care experiences? If so, can you get your hands on that satisfaction data to see how specific doctors and claims-handling processes measure up? Not a big deal, but nice to have.

☛ Are Spanish- or other language-speaking reps and nurses offered, if that's an issue for you?

Ill-advised Insurance Office

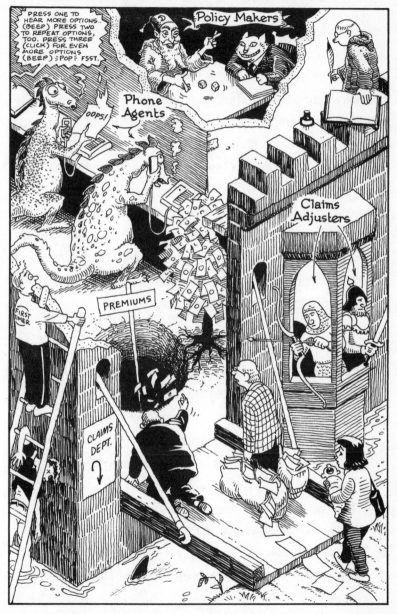

How Healthy Is This Plan?

Once you know your company is solid, apply your detective powers to carefully reviewing the specific insurance policy you're buying. Don't assume the policy is adequate because you have confidence in the company; every policy is different, and if the wording in yours leaves you without a pot to . . . cook in, the caliber of the company may not mean a thing. (You signed on the dotted line, didn't you?) One terrible bit of news: To make sure you know the ins and outs of your policy, you need to read that entire insufferably boring booklet with all the policy rules and limits and bylaws and heretofores and therewiths. Get it from your HR department or the insurer. If it makes it more enjoyable, read it aloud and set it to song. To give your policy the third degree, ask:

☞ What hospitals and doctors are in the plan's network? Duh, right? Are the hospitals Joint Commission–accredited? Check this again, to make sure that the Dr. Frank you circled in the book is indeed *your* Dr. Frank. If your doctor isn't in the network, ask your HR department to twist the insurer's arm to add him. Also ask your doc to consider joining the insurer's network.

☞ What's not covered? These are called exclusions.

☞ Will I have continued care on my preexisting conditions?

☞ What will happen if I get cancer, get pregnant, or become disabled? These are the biggies that really test insurance coverage.

- ☛ Can I use an out-of-network doctor, and what will it cost? Hopefully you can, and the plan will pay 80 percent of the cost after the deductible.
- ☛ What percentage of the total cost will I pay for common services and diagnostic procedures, such as X-rays or blood tests?
- ☛ If I get extremely sick, how much freedom does my doctor have in coordinating care, and can I see any specialist at all?
- ☛ How much will the plan pay for generic and brand-name prescription drugs?
- ☛ Can I increase my deductible and pay lower premiums?

X-Ray Tech

- ☛ What's the yearly out-of-pocket limit? A typical figure is $2,000.
- ☛ What's the maximum lifetime benefit? It should be at least $5 million.
- ☛ What is the coverage for mental health?
- ☛ What's the coverage for alternative therapies, such as chiropractic and acupuncture?
- ☛ Will follow-up care, such as nursing-home or home-health care, be covered?
- ☛ If I have a serious medical problem, will the plan provide someone to oversee care and make sure my needs are met?
- ☛ Which specific conditions or injuries does the plan deem as emergencies requiring urgent care? You need to know this,

because if you take an ambulance to the ER for something the policy considers nonurgent, you might foot the entire bill. See the sidebar "Forget About Finding My Arm, Just Call the Claims Hotline!" on page 327.

☛ Does the plan have a high-deductible version? See the sidebar below.

☛ At what age will my children be cut off from the plan? Will it be eighteen or twenty-one or twenty-five? (Use this tidbit to get their bottoms out of the house!)

☛ If I'm in a foreign country and have an emergency, will this plan pay to evacuate me at my request? This one isn't a must, but it's a nice bonus. (Mention that you're accustomed to flying first class. Can't hurt, right?)

GOD BLESS THE HSA

Health savings accounts are another fairly new wrinkle in the nation's health care arsenal. If you select an insurance plan that has a high deductible (say, $1,000 or more, instead of the usual $250 or $500) that you have to pay out of your pocket before coverage kicks in, you can open a health savings account to pay for those medical costs—and to also save money for future medical expenses. (Yes, you can use it only for health care expenses, so the Aruba trip might not cut it.) The government doesn't tax the contributions or the interest in this savings account, so the cash can build quickly. Best of all, you can't lose the account. Regardless of whether you purchased the high-deductible insurance plan through your employer or a private policy on your own, your health savings account remains yours and yours alone. You can even keep it if you move to another state. And it doesn't have the infamous catch that comes with other types of medical-spending accounts: you don't forfeit unused HSA funds at the end of the year or in the following spring.

You Will Not Be Denied

D-E-N-I-E-D.

That word brings us back to our dating years. And it's also one that people really dislike seeing stamped on a piece of important correspondence, like a parole application. Or worse, a health-insurance claim. That's because each one of the six letters could represent tens of thousands of bucks that the folks at the insurance company are saying—nay, declaring—is your responsibility to pay, not theirs. Even if it's only a few hundred dollars, it's still a massive bummer when you were expecting to rip open a check for that amount.

You can fight the system. And you can win.

If you've ever fought to reverse an insurance-claim denial in the past, you'll have fond memories that make our warning sound like the understatement it is: you'll need persistence, patience, frustration-coping ability, persistence, and attention to detail. And persistence. Mix all those with another healthy dose of persistence, and there's a better-than-not chance that you'll shake those dollars out of your insurer. A study by the

Rand Corporation, an esteemed nonprofit research group, found that patients who appealed denied insurance claims were successful in getting their cash in far more than half the cases—and in more than 90 percent of the denials involving emergency care! It's amazing that only a small fraction of patients appeal denied claims. Clearly insurance companies intimidate many people into accepting a no, and they're good at that. But for the Smart Patients who persist (and we'll vouch that they never run from a fight), insurance companies eventually fold like a lousy poker hand. So when you're dealing with your insurer, emulate Agatha Christie's Miss Marple: Be dogged and persistent and don't be afraid to take your question to the top brass, but be polite enough so that no one slams the phone down on you.

Miss Marple

When your insurer refuses to pay a claim you believe is legit, take these tenacious tips to speak its language and speed its reversal.

Know the Company's Agenda

Remember, insurance companies aren't making decisions based on giving you personally the best care possible; they're making the best average decisions that will be workable for most patients. These decisions become standard policy, and they don't like to deviate from their standard policy for anybody. One-size-fits-all coverage is a lot easier for them. Your goal is to get them to forget about their standard policy and to deal with you as an individual.

Remember, No Doesn't Mean No

It means try again until your gums start bleeding. But pick your battles; don't fight them to cover a treatment that's not FDA approved because they probably won't bend.

Learn the Technical Reason Your Claim Has Been Refused

It may be something like "the prescribed dosage exceeds standard guidelines." This gives you a specific target to attack.

Consider Committing the Crime First

Statistically, it's easier to get forgiveness than permission. The Rand study found that while patients won their appeals in half the cases in which they had already paid for the medical treatment, those who were trying to get the insurer to pay for an upcoming treatment were successful only 36 percent of the time. Naturally, this is a gamble, but the odds are a little more in your favor when you're seeking reimbursement.

Go Head-to-Head with the Plan Rep

The customer-service rep who answers the 800 number is your first potential ally, so try to persuade that rep to help before you launch a formal appeal. Get the names and phone numbers of every rep you speak with. If your insurer has nurse case managers, ask to work directly with one of them. Bring your doctor on board in proving why the insurance company's technical reason for denying the claim is wrong. As you're doing this, make sure that you don't exceed the deadline to file an appeal, if the insurer has one. Some give you thirty or forty-five days after the claim denial to appeal.

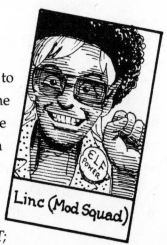

Telephone Operator

Pull the Trigger

You've gotten nowhere? It's time to formally appeal. This is not the time to be meek; assert yourself and make your voice heard (think Linc from *The Mod Squad*). Ask the insurer and your HR department at work to send you the complete rules for filing an appeal. Follow them to the *T;*

Linc (Mod Squad)

the insurance company is hoping you'll flub something or send in incomplete paperwork so it can toss your appeal without any sweat. Do you need to get a second opinion? Which bills, test results, or other paperwork do you need to include in your appeal application? Be exacting. For info sources to help you craft your appeal, see the Web site at **www.patients arepowerful.org.** If you're appealing a Medicare denial, tap the knowledge from the Medicare Rights Center at **www.medi carerights.org,** 888-466-9050 (for people appealing an HMO decision) or 202-589-1316.

Bombard Them with Facts

You won't get anywhere with passionate pleas. You need lab data, national trend info, physician letters, and other hard records to show the insurer why it has no basis to deny your claim. Ask your doc to send a letter saying why you need the treatment; it'll pack more punch coming from him or her.

Seek the MD

Your goal is to get your case to the insurer's medical director or staff doctor. A doctor will usually look at your situation with more sympathetic eyes and give more clout to good patient care versus follow-

Insco Staff Doctor

ing the standard policies. Keep pushing until you get a clinician.

Use Smart Patient Timing

When you get to that doc, you want to speak to him or her on a Monday morning or a Friday afternoon, when he's likely in the best mood.

You can't reach the doctor? Unacceptable! Tell the insurer that you're going to bring the matter to the state department of insurance or the attorney general. Don't use this threat too soon; it will cost you goodwill (which still influences some folks on this good earth, believe it or not), so save it as a last resort.

Rat 'Em Out

No satisfaction, even when the doctor gets involved? If you're not ready to say uncle yet (did we mention something about persistence?), take your appeal to the state department of insurance.

We're pulling for you.

Appendix 1
Medical Jargon Explained

From talking to your doctor, watching television, reading novels and magazine articles—maybe even playing doctor as a kid—we're sure you're familiar with hundreds of common and even technical medical terms that doctors, nurses and other health care workers throw around. But rest assured there are thousands that never make it into TV scripts or popular use, and we still had to learn 'em all. There are new ones to learn all the time. So you'll never feel like an outsider (and no Smart Patient does), use this reference glossary to get plain-English translations of terms your doctor uses—or you overhear in the hospital cafeteria—every day. You'll find more definitions at the Web site **www.medterms.com.**

Acute: refers to a medical problem that requires immediate attention. (For example, "By the way she came at me with that needle, you would think it was an acute problem." We may also hear a patient say, "That resident was acute," but they mean something else.)
Ad lib: at liberty; not referring to a fugitive, but to your freedom to do or not do something as you wish. ("Patient can now resume exercising *ad lib*.")

Algia: when used in a word, it means "pain" or "ache." (For example, *myalgia* means muscle pain because *my* means muscle; never used metaphorically, such as "That insurance company is a real algia in the neck.")

Allergy: when your immune system overreacts to a normally harmless substance such as pollen, dust, or certain foods.

AMI: acute myocardial infarction, aka heart attack.

Bacteria: the one-celled microorganisms found in air, water, and soil that can cause infectious diseases.

Benign: when used in reference to tumors, it means not harmful or noncancerous; also used to describe people.

Beta blockers: a class of drugs used to treat high blood pressure by slowing the heart rate; also used for stage fright.

C/O: the patient's concern, the problem he's complaining about.

CABG: coronary artery bypass grafting, pronounced like *cabbage*. Saying "Your father was just a simple CABG" is not an insult.

Cardiac arrest: when the heart stops beating; bad problem.

Cardio: when used as part of a word, refers to the heart. (For example, "I detest cardio exercise" means you hate exercise that makes you break a sweat and strengthens the heart.)

Catheter: A tube that's inserted into the bladder to allow continuous urination into a container. (Yes, there are more pleasant things in the world.) Also called a "Foley," after the name of the urologist who invented it, Frederick Foley.

CBC: abbreviation for complete blood cell count.

Chronic: an ongoing condition that can be controlled but not cured, such as diabetes, asthma, or hypertension (unlike an acute condition, which requires immediate treatment).

Code blue or code red: A patient requires CPR (cardiopulmonary resuscitation) to save her life. Patients should avoid being involved in these.

Code pink: Nurses might announce this code if a doctor is speaking in a rude manner to one of them, which will alert other nurses to gather around their colleague and stare at the doctor, which usually ends the rudeness pretty quickly.

Cognitive dysfunction: used to refer to patients who have medical conditions that cloud their thinking, but doctors also sometimes use this to describe one another.

Compliant: how cooperative the person is. (For example, "Like many Americans, that patient was poorly compliant in taking his medications.")

Contraindication: a condition that makes a particular treatment or procedure inadvisable. (For example, "You'd be unwise to proceed on this contraindicated operation.")

D/C: discharge, or to discontinue, as in "patient was DC'ed on April 2."

Degenerative disorder: a condition that causes body parts to deteriorate over time, such as muscular dystrophy or arthritis or aging.

Derm or derma: when used as part of a word, refers to skin.

Diagnosis: the process of identifying a condition or disease (what you've got, hopefully).

Differential diagnosis: list of different conditions that can cause the symptoms a patient is experiencing.

Dis: when used as part of a word, it means removal (such as disability); also used as slang as short for disrespect ("Yo, did you just dis me?").

Dys: when used as part of a word, it means difficulty—such as, "He is a dysfunctional person."

Ecto: when used as part of a word, means outside or external. (For example, an ectopic pregnancy develops outside the uterus.)

Edema: abnormal buildup of fluid that causes swelling.

EEG: abbreviation for electroencephalogram, a test that measures the brain's electrical activity. (Urbanites insult each other by insisting that they have a flat line or no activity on their EEG.)

EKG: sometimes called ECG, the abbreviation for electrocardiogram, a diagnostic test that shows the heart's electrical activity.

Electrolytes: chemical substances in the body that conduct electricity and are routinely checked on blood tests because they are clues to numerous problems.

Embolism: when a blood vessel is blocked, such as by a blood clot, air bubble, or foreign object.

Endo: when used as part of a word, means inward or internal. (For example, the endocranium is the membrane that lines the inside of the skull.)

Epidermis: the outer layer of skin.

Fascinoma: not an actual disease but rather slang for any fascinating case; something the doctors don't see often.

Foley: *see* catheter.

Gastri or gastro: when used as part of a word, refers to the stomach or abdomen.

GI series: tests, usually X-rays, of the digestive system.

HA: headache.

HBD: abbreviation for has been drinking. (Anybody in the middle of a double shift or a busy day may describe themselves as WRBD, or would rather be drinking.)

Hema or hemo: when used as part of word, means blood.

Hyper: when used as part of a word means above or beyond. (For example, hyperglycemia means abnormally high blood sugar level; hypertension means abnormally high blood pressure; hyperthyroidism refers to a condition in which the thyroid gland produces excess levels of thyroid hormone, and hyperactive refers to many children who don't want to go to bed.)

Hyperglycemia: abnormally high blood-sugar level.

Hypertension: abnormally high blood pressure.

Hypo: when used as part of a word means under or below. (For example, hypoglycemia means abnormally low blood sugar, and hypotension means low blood pressure.)

In vitro: occurring in an artificial environment (such as with in vitro fertilization, which occurs outside the human body).

Indication: the condition that requires a specific treatment or procedure. (For example, "Why is my tumor an indication to use this particular surgical technique?")

Intra: inside or within. (For example, intracellular functions occur within a cell.)

Intravenous (IV): inserted into your vein.

Itis: when used in a word, means inflammation (for example, gastritis occurs when the stomach lining is inflamed); not used to describe inflammatory people.

IV drip: An intravenous tube (like the one that goes in your arm) that administers medication or a fluid into your body one drip at a time; also a term for an overeducated, boring person.

Lipo: when used as part of a word, means fat. (For example, liposuction refers to the removal of fat from the body.)

Malignant: dangerous to health; also used to refer to malevolent people.

Membrane: a thin layer of tissue that covers or lines part of your body.

Metastasis: when cancer cells spread beyond the site where the cancer originated.

Minor surgery: usually refers to surgery performed without general anesthesia (meaning you remain awake) or surgery performed on somebody else. (Surgery performed on *you* is rarely considered minor.)

MI: stands for myocardial infarction, which describes the damage that occurs to the heart due to a decrease in blood flow; commonly called heart attack.

My, myo: when used as part of a word, refers to muscle. (Mycology is the branch of physiology that studies muscles.)

Myopia: nearsightedness; often an accurate description of a bothersome relative.

Narcotic: a drug that will dull your senses, usually to put you to sleep or to kill pain. If patients hear someone say, "We'll administer narcotics," they often freak out, thinking that we're going to hand them a crack pipe or otherwise give them a dangerously addictive drug, illicit or not. Relax; *narcotic* was a medical word long before it became sullied on the street, and we're not giving it up. Sometimes, narcotics are just what the doctor ordered.

Nephr, nepho: when used as part of a word, refers to the kidneys. (Nephrology is the branch of medicine that studies kidneys and kidney disorders.)

Neuro: when used as part of a word, it refers to the nervous system including the brain. (A neurologist, sometimes called a brain doctor, studies the nervous system.)

Noninvasive: a treatment or technique that doesn't enter the body.

Nouveau: sounds a bit like neuro, but it's a French word that's being used to described a lot of fancy, overpriced restaurant food.

NPO: *nil per os,* or the patient should take "nothing by mouth," foot included.

Onco: when used as part of a word, means tumor or mass. (An oncologist studies tumors, some of which are cancerous.)

Osis: when used at the end of a word, means condition or disease. (It's not a goddess.)

Osteo: when used as part of a word, means bone.

Palpation: technique of using hands to help make a diagnosis.

Palpitation: condition when the heart pounds or races; often happens when falling in love, which should not be confused with a form of palpation.

Phlebo: when used as part of a word, refers to veins. (For example, a phlebotomist takes blood from a vein.)

Plegia: when used as part of a word, means paralysis (such as paraplegia).

Post: when used as part of a word, means after. (For example, "How important is it to avoid this food during the postoperative period?")

PRN: take the pill or the therapy as needed.

Prognosis: the likely course of a disease or condition.

Reflex: your body's involuntary movement in response to a stimulus.

Renal failure: the inability of your body's kidneys to function.

Sangui or sanguin: when used as part of a word, refers to blood.

Sarco: when used as part of a word, refers to flesh.

Sepsis: bacterial infection in the blood.

Sign: evidence of a disease or medical condition observed by someone else, such as by your doctor (as opposed to a symptom which is observed by the patient).

Stat: urgent, right away ("Doctor Smith to Room 142, stat!").

Static: a stat situation that hasn't changed or been resolved. Also what you get when your actions cause friction.

Stroke: when the blood supply to a section of the brain is completely blocked and causes loss of or diminished sensation, inability to move a body part, or loss of consciousness.

Sub: when used as part of a word, means under or less than. For example, "I was subverted in my attempt to extract the subcutaneous splinter by suboptimal operative conditions."

Symptom: when a patient reports evidence of a disease or medical condition (as opposed to a sign, which is observed by a doctor or other person).

Syndrome: a group of signs and symptoms that occur at the same time and are associated with a particular condition.

Tachy: when used as part of a word, means fast or rapid. (Tachycardia is an abnormally fast heartbeat.)

Thermo: when used as part of a word, refers to heat; does not refer to underwear.

Tissue: a group of cells that work together to perform a particular function; and the box of nose wipes on the bedside table.

Topical: pertaining to the surface of a body part (such as with a topical medication, which is applied directly to the skin).

Tumor: a solid mass that grows from normal body parts or tissue. ("Tumor" is a scary word, but most tumors aren't cancerous.)

Ulcer: lesion in a part of the body caused by infection or disease.

Uro, urono: when used as part of a word, refers to the urine or urinary tract.

Vaccine: a substance created from weakened or dead bacteria or viruses that is used to stimulate the body's immune defense to that substance.

Virus: a microorganism that can live only by attaching itself to a living cell and which can cause diseases. (The common cold, measles, and chicken pox are all caused by viruses.)

WNL: means within normal limits, as opposed to we never looked.

Workup: an intensive diagnostic study.

Xeno: when used as part of a word, means foreign.

Appendix 2
Sample Forms

Your Health Journal

 ## THE BASICS

Name: _____

Height: _____

Weight: _____

Date of birth: _____

Primary doctor: _____

   Contact info: _____

Specialist: _____

   Contact info: _____

Specialist: _____

   Contact info: _____

Specialist: _____

   Contact info: _____

Specialist: _____

   Contact info: _____

Pharmacy: _____

   Contact info: _____

Health insurance: _____

   Policy number: _____

   Contact info: _____

Vision insurance: _____

   Policy number: _____

   Contact info: _____

Dental insurance: _____

   Policy number: _____

   Contact info: _____

Social Security Number: _____

Blood Type: _____

Date of last physical exam: _____

Medication allergies: _____

YOUR HEALTH NOW

Existing Conditions

Write down every SIGNIFICANT ailment or condition that you have RIGHT NOW.

Ailment/Condition	Current treatment or current medication you're taking for it (include name, dosage, and frequency)	Other info (name of specialist, surgery type and date, etc.)

Current Health

✔ Are any specific health conditions/symptoms bothering you? What are the symptoms? When did they start?

✔ Are you on a special or restricted diet?

✔ Are you under medical care? For what?

Current Medications

(Prescribed meds, herbal supplements, vitamins, over-the-counter drugs—everything that you are taking on a regular basis for any reason at all)

Name of medication	Dosage and frequency	Date you began taking it	The reason you're taking it	Prescribing physician (with contact info)	Special instructions (e.g., take with liquid or food)

Current Medical Symptoms

Context and length of illness can often be important clues, and many patients don't think to really record when things start and how they feel.

Date	Description of symptoms (include timing, duration, location, intensity, and provoking events)	Action

Vital Statistics/Lab Numbers

These numbers are an important part of understanding your overall health. Ask your doctor to help you keep track of them.

Date	Ht	Wt	Blood Pres	Heart Rate	HDL	LDL	Total Chol	Trig	Blood Sugar	CRP	HCT

Ht, height; wt, weight; Blood Pres, blood pressure; HDL, high-density lipoprotein; LDL, low-density lipoprotein; Total Chol, total cholesterol; Trig, triglycerides; CRP, C-reactive protein; HCT, hematocrit.

Immunizations

Fill in date received and any followup needed.

Tetanus, Diphtheria (td): _____

Influenza (Flu shot): _____

Hepatitis B: _____

Hepatitis A: _____

Measles, Mumps, Rubella: _____

Meningococcus (Meningitis): _____

Chicken Pox: _____

Pneumonia (Pneumococcal): _____

TB Screen: _____

Other: _____

Major Illnesses

Date	Illness Type	Treatment

Hospitalizations

Date	Reason	Treatment

Surgeries/Procedures

Date	Type	Outcome

Chronic Diseases

Type	When diagnosed	Treatment	Current treatment

Allergies/reactions (e.g., medications, latex):

_____

_____

Physical limitations (e.g., corrected vision, hearing aid, arthritis):

_____

_____

YOUR FAMILY HISTORY

Relevant Family Health History

List the significant ailments and conditions experienced by family members and relatives, back to your grandparents, that your physician feels are a GENETIC CONCERN. Include your spouse, but the rest of the list should be blood relatives.

Relative (how related to you)	Condition or ailment	Age (or date of death and age attained)	How it was treated	If deceased, did it cause or seriously contribute to death?

 KEEPING UP WITH YOUR HEALTH

Health Exams and Screenings

Fill in the date that the test is performed and the results. Make several copies of the form so you can use it for several years.

	Date	Results
Urinalysis		
Eye exam		
Blood pressure		
Cholesterol		
Depression		
STDs		
Colon exam		
Skin exam		
Mammogram		
Pelvic exam		
Pap test		
Testicular exam		

In Case of Emergency (ICE)

Who should be called in case of an emergency? Do you have any legal documents or directives about your care?

Main Contact

Name: _____

Relationship: _____

Address: _____

Home phone: _____

Work phone: _____

Cell phone: _____

Secondary Contact

Name: _____

Relationship: _____

Address: _____

Home phone: _____

Work phone: _____

Cell phone: _____

Organ Donor   Yes _____   No _____

Living Will   Yes _____   No _____

Location: _____

Do-Not-Resuscitate Order   Yes _____   No _____

Location: _____

Health care Proxy   Yes _____   No _____

Location: _____

Contact: _____

Medical Power of Attorney   Yes _____   No _____

Location: _____

Contact: _____

APPENDIX 2

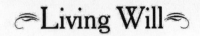 Living Will

DECLARATION

This declaration is made this _____ day of _____ (month, year).

I, _____ , being of sound mind, willfully and voluntarily make known my desires that my moment of death shall not be artificially postponed.

If at any time I should have an incurable and irreversible injury, disease, or illness judged to be a terminal condition by my attending physician who has personally examined me and has determined that my death is imminent except for death delaying procedures, I direct that such procedures which would only prolong the dying process be withheld or withdrawn, and that I be permitted to die naturally with only the administration of medication, sustenance, or the performance of any medical procedure deemed necessary by my attending physician to provide me with comfort care.

In the absence of my ability to give directions regarding the use of such death delaying procedures, it is my intention that this declaration shall be honored by my family and physician as the final expression of my legal right to refuse medical or surgical treatment and accept the consequences from such refusal.

Signed _____

City, County and State of Residence _____

The declarant is personally known to me and I believe him or her to be of sound mind. I saw the declarant sign the declaration in my presence (or the declarant acknowledged in my presence that he or she had signed the declaration) and I signed the declaration as a witness in the presence of the declarant. I did not sign the declarant's signature above for or at the direction of the declarant. At the date of this instrument, I am not entitled to any portion of the estate of the declarant according to the laws of intestate succession or, to the best of my knowledge and belief, under any will of declarant or other instrument taking effect at declarant's death, or directly financially responsible for declarant's medical care.

Witness _____

Witness _____

Illinois Statutory Short Form
⌐Power of Attorney for Health Care⌐

(NOTICE: the purpose of this power of attorney is to give the person you designate (your "agent") broad powers to make health care decisions for you, including power to require, consent to or withdraw any type of personal care or medical treatment for any physical or mental condition and to admit you to or discharge you from any hospital, home or other institution. This form does not impose a duty on your agent to exercise granted powers; but when powers are exercised, your agent will have to use due care to act for your benefit and in accordance with this form and keep a record of receipts, disbursements and significant actions taken as agent. A court can take away powers of your agent if it finds the agent is not acting properly. You may name successor agents under this form but not co-agents, and no health care provider may be named. Unless you expressly limit the duration of this power in the manner provided below, until you revoke this power or a court acting on your behalf terminates it, your agent may exercise the powers given here throughout your lifetime, even after you become disabled. The powers you give your agent, your right to revoke those powers and the penalties for violating the law are explained more fully in sections 4-5, 4-6, 4-9 and 4-10(b) of the Illinois "Powers of Attorney for Health Care Law" of which this form is a part. That law expressly permits the use of any different form of power of attorney you may desire. If there is anything about this form that you do not understand, you should ask a lawyer to explain it to you.)

POWER OF ATTORNEY made this _____ day of _____ (month, year).

1. I, _____

(insert name and address of principal)

hereby appoint: _____

(insert name and address of agent)

as my attorney-in-fact (my "agent") to act for me and in my name (in any way I could act in person) to make any and all decisions for me concerning my personal care, medical treatment, hospitalization and health care and to require, withhold or withdraw any type of medical treatment or procedure, even though my death may ensue. My agent shall have the same access to my medical records that I have, including the right to disclose the contents to others. My agent shall also have full power to authorize an autopsy and direct the disposition of my remains. Effective upon my death, my agent has the full power to make an anatomical gift of the following (initial one):

Any organ:
Specific organs:

(The above grant of power is intended to be as broad as possible so that your agent will have authority to make any decision you could make to obtain or terminate any type of health care, including withdrawal of food and water and other life-sustaining measures, if your agent believes such action would be consistent with your intent and desires. If you wish to limit the scope of your agent's powers or prescribe special rules or limit the power to make an anatomical gift, authorize autopsy or dispose of remains, you may do so in the following paragraphs.)

2. The powers granted above shall not include the following powers or shall be subject to the following rules or limitations (here you may include any specific limitations you deem appropriate, such as: your own definition of when life-sustaining measures should be withheld; a direction to continue food and fluids or life-sustaining treatment in all events; or instructions to refuse any specific types of treatment that are inconsistent with your religious beliefs or unacceptable to you for any other reason, such as blood transfusion, electro-convulsive therapy, amputation, psychosurgery, voluntary admission to a mental institution, etc.):

_____

_____

_____

_____

(continued)

APPENDIX 2

(The subject of life-sustaining treatment is of particular importance. For your convenience in dealing with that subject, some general statements concerning the withholding or removal of life-sustaining treatment are set forth below. If you agree with one of these statements, you may initial that statement; but do not initial more than one):

<u>Initialed</u>   I do not want my life to be prolonged nor do I want life-sustaining treatment to be provided or continued if my agent believes the burdens of the treatment outweigh the expected benefits. I want my agent to consider the relief of suffering, the expense involved and the quality as well as the possible extension of my life in making decisions concerning life-sustaining treatment.

<u>Initialed</u>   I want my life to be prolonged and I want life-sustaining treatment to be provided or continued unless I am in a coma which my attending physician believes to be irreversible, in accordance with reasonable medical standards at the time of reference. If and when I have suffered irreversible coma, I want life-sustaining treatment to be withheld or discontinued.

<u>Initialed</u>   I want my life to be prolonged to the greatest extent possible without regard to my condition, the chances I have for recovery or the cost of the procedures.

(This power of attorney may be amended or revoked by you in the manner provided in section 4-6 of the Illinois "powers of attorney for health care law" (see the back of this form). Absent amendment or revocation, the authority granted in this power of attorney will become effective at the time this power is signed and will continue until your death, and beyond if anatomical gift, autopsy or disposition of remains is authorized, unless a limitation on the beginning date or duration is made by initialing and completing either or both of the following:)

3.( ) This power of attorney shall become effective on _____

_____
(insert a future date or event during your lifetime, such as court determination of your disability, when you want this power to first take effect)

4.( ) This power of attorney shall terminate on _____

_____
(insert a future date or event, such as court determination of your disability, when you want this power to terminate prior to your death)

(If you wish to name successor agents, insert the names and addresses of such successors in the following paragraph.)

5. If any agent named by me shall die, become incompetent, resign, refuse to accept the office of agent or be unavailable, I name the following (each to act alone and successively, in the order named) as successors to such agent:

_____

_____

_____

_____

For purposes of this paragraph 5, a person shall be considered to be incompetent if and while the person is a minor or an adjudicated incompetent or disabled person or the person is unable to give prompt and intelligent consideration to health care matters, as certified by a licensed physician.

(continued)

(If you wish to name your agent as guardian of your person, in the event a court decides that one should be appointed, you may, but are not required to, do so by retaining the following paragraph. The court will appoint your agent if the court finds that such appointment will serve your best interests and welfare. Strike out paragraph 6 if you do not want your agent to act as guardian.)

6. If a guardian of my person is to be appointed, I nominate the agent acting under this power of attorney as such guardian, to serve without bond or security.

7. I am fully informed as to all the contents of this form and understand the full import of this grant of powers to my agent.

Signed _____

(principal)

The principal has had an opportunity to read the above form and has signed the form or acknowledged his or her signature or mark on the form in my presence.

_____ Residing at _____

(witness)

(You may, but are not required to, request your agent and successor agents to provide specimen signatures below. If you include specimen signatures in this power of attorney, you must complete the certification opposite the signatures of the agents.)

Specimen signatures of agent (and successors)   I certify that the signatures of my agent (and successors) are correct.

_____   _____

(agent)   (principal)

_____   _____

(successor agent)   (principal)

_____   _____

(successor agent)   (principal)

APPENDIX 2

State of Illinois
Do Not Resuscitate (DNR) Order

I, _____, (print full name) **DO NOT AUTHORIZE CARDIOPULMONARY RESUSCITATION.**
I (or my legal representative) understand that this order remains in effect until revoked by me (or my legal representative) or
the attending physician. I (or my legal representative) acknowledge that cardiopulmonary resuscitation (CPR) will not be performed if breathing or heart beat stops. (The signatures of [a] the patient **OR** legal representative, [b] the physician and
[c] two witnesses are required.)

Printed name of patient	Signature of patient	Date
Printed name of physician	Signature of physician	Date
Effective date		
Printed name of witness	Signature of witness	Date
Address of witness		
Printed name of witness	Signature of witness	Date
Address of witness		

Legal Representative's Signature of Consent for Patient Lacking Decision Making Capacity
(If the patient lacks decision making capacity, then a signature in this section is required.)

Printed name of (circle appropriate title) legal guardian
OR durable power of attorney for health care agent
OR surrogate decision maker

Street Address

City, State, ZIP

Signature of legal representative

Date

Illinois Department of Public Health
535 W. Jefferson St.
Springfield, IL 62761
217-785-2080,
TTY (hearing impaired use only)
800-547-0466

Reproduce on brightly colored orange paper

Appendix 3

Resources

Find a Board-Certified Doctor

Want to know whether a doctor is board certified in a particular area? Contact one or more of the twenty-four boards of the American Board of Medical Specialties to get referrals for board-certified doctors, or to find out if a doctor is board certified in a particular specialty.

Allergy and Immunology
510 Walnut Street
Suite 1701
Philadelphia, PA 19106-3699
1-866-264-5568
www.abai.org

Anesthesiology
4101 Lake Boone Trail
Suite 510

Raleigh, NC 27607-7506
919-881-2570
www.theaba.org

Colon and Rectal Surgery
20600 Eureka Road
Suite 600
Taylor, MI 48180
734-282-9400
www.abcrs.org

Dermatology
Henry Ford Health System
1 Ford Place
Detroit, MI 48202-3450
313-874-1088
www.abderm.org

Emergency Medicine
3000 Coolidge Road
East Lansing, MI 48823-6319
517-332-4800
www.abem.org/public

Family Medicine
2228 Young Drive
Lexington, KY 40505-4294
859-269-5626
www.theabfm.org

Internal Medicine
510 Walnut Street
Suite 1700
Philadelphia, PA 19106-3699
800-441-2246
www.abim.org

Medical Genetics
9650 Rockville Pike
Bethesda, MD 20814-3998
301-634-7315
www.abmg.org

Neurological Surgery
Smith Tower
Suite 2139
6550 Fannin Street
Houston, TX 77030-2701
713-441-6015
www.abns.org

Nuclear Medicine
4555 Forest Park Boulevard
Suite 119
St. Louis, MO 63108
314-367-2225
www.abnm.org

Obstetrics and Gynecology
2915 Vine Street
Suite 300
Dallas, TX 75204
214-871-1619
www.abog.org

Ophthalmology
111 Presidential Boulevard
Suite 241
Bala Cynwyd, PA 19004-1075
610-664-1175
www.abop.org

Orthopaedic Surgery
400 Silver Cedar Court
Chapel Hill, NC 27514
919-929-7103
www.abos.org

Otolaryngology
5615 Kirby Drive
Suite 600
Houston, TX 77005
713-850-0399
www.aboto.org

Pathology
PO Box 25915
Tampa, FL 33622-5915
813-286-2444
www.abpath.org

Pediatrics
111 Silver Cedar Court
Chapel Hill, NC 27514-1651
919-929-0461
www.abp.org

Physical Medicine and
 Rehabilitation
3015 Allegro Park Lane SW
Rochester, MN 55902-4139
507-282-1776
www.abpmr.org

Plastic Surgery
Seven Penn Center
Suite 400
1635 Market Street
Philadelphia, PA 19103-2204
215-587-9322
www.abplsurg.org

Preventive Medicine
330 South Wells Street
Suite 1018
Chicago, IL 60606-7106
312-939-2276
www.abprevmed.org

Psychiatry and Neurology
500 Lake Cook Road
Suite 335
Deerfield, IL 60015-5249
847-945-7900
www.abpn.com

Radiology
5441 East Williams Boulevard
Suite 200
Tucson, AZ 85711
520-790-2900
www.theabr.org

Surgery
1617 John F. Kennedy Boulevard
Suite 860
Philadelphia, PA 19103-1847
215-568-4000
www.absurgery.org

Urology
2216 Ivy Road
Suite 210
Charlottesville, VA 22903
434-979-0059
www.abu.org

Thoracic Surgery
633 North St. Clair Street
Suite 2320
Chicago, IL 60611
312-202-5900
www.abts.org

Medical Licensing Boards

Contact the medical licensing board or the board of osteopathic medicine in the state in which he or she practices. (Osteopaths are licensed physicians who focus on preventive health care and receive extra training in the musculoskeletal system.) Ask whether the doctor is licensed, and whether the board has ever taken disciplinary action against him or her. If it has, you can request a copy of the disciplinary order.

Alabama State Board of Medical
   Examiners
PO Box 946
Montgomery, AL 36101-0946

800-227-2606
Fax: 334-242-4155
www.albme.org

Alaska State Medical Board
550 West Seventh Avenue
Suite 1500
Anchorage, AK 99501-3567
907-269-8163
Fax: 907-269-8196
www.dced.state.ak.us/occ/
   pmed.htm

Arizona Medical Board
9545 East Doubletree Ranch
   Road
Scottsdale, AZ 85258-5514
877-255-2212
Fax: 480-551-2704
www.azmdboard.org

Arizona Board of Osteopathic
   Examiners in Medicine and
   Surgery
9535 East Doubletree Ranch
   Road
Scottsdale, AZ 85258-5539
480-657-7703
Fax: 480-657-7715
www.azosteoboard.org

Arkansas State Medical Board
2100 Riverfront Drive
Suite 220

Little Rock, AR 72202-1793
501-296-1802
Fax: 501-603-3555
www.armedicalboard.org

Medical Board of California
1426 Howe Avenue
Suite 54
Sacramento, CA 95825-3236
916-263-2382
Fax: 916-263-2944
www.medbd.ca.gov

Osteopathic Medical Board of
   California
2720 Gateway Oaks Drive
Suite 350
Sacramento, CA 95833-3500
916-263-3100
www.ombc.ca.gov

Colorado Board of Medical
   Examiners
1560 Broadway
Suite 1300
Denver, CO 80202-5140
303-894-7690
Fax: 303-894-7692
www.dora.state.co.us/medical

Connecticut Medical Examining
Board
PO Box 340308
Hartford, CT 06134-0308
860/509-7648
Licensing information: 860-509-
7563
Fax: 860-509-7553
www.dph.state.ct.us

Delaware Board of Medical
Practice
PO Box 1401
Dover, DE 19903
302-744-4507
Fax: 302-739-2711
www.professionallicensing.state
.de.us

District of Columbia Board of
Medicine
717 14th Street NW
Suite 600
Washington, DC 20010
202-724-4900
Fax: 202-442-9431
dchealth.dc.gov

Florida Board of Medicine
Department of Health

4052 Bald Cypress Way
BIN #C03
Tallahassee, FL 32399-3253
850-245-4131
www.doh.state.fl.us

Florida Board of Osteopathic
Medicine
4052 Bald Cypress Way
BIN #C06
Tallahassee, FL 32399-1753
850-245-4161
Fax: 850-487-9874
www.doh.state.fl.us/mqa/
osteopath

Georgia Composite State Board
of Medical Examiners
2 Peachtree Street NW
36th Floor
Atlanta, GA 30303-3465
404-656-3913
Fax: 404-656-9723
www.medicalboard.state.ga.us

Hawaii Board of Medical
Examiners Department of
Commerce and Consumer
Affairs
PO Box 3469

Honolulu, HI 96813
808-586-3000
www.hawaii.gov/dcca/
    areas/pvl

Idaho State Board of Medicine
1755 Westgate Drive
Suite 140
Boise, ID 83720
208-327-7000
Fax: 208-327-7005
www.bom.state.id.us

Illinois Department of
    Financial & Professional
    Regulation
James R. Thompson Center
100 West Randolph Street
Suite 9-300
Chicago, IL 60601
312-814-6910
www.idfpr.com

Illinois Department of
    Professional
    Regulation/Licensure
320 West Washington Street
3rd Floor
Springfield, IL 62786
217-785-0800

Fax: 217-524-2169
www.dpr.state.il.us

Indiana Professional Licensing
    Agency
402 West Washington Street
Room W072
Indianapolis, IN 46204
317-234-2060
Fax: 317-233-4236
www.in.gov/hpb

Iowa Board of Medical
    Examiners
400 SW Eighth Street
Suite C
Des Moines, IA 50309-4686
515-281-5171
Fax: 515-242-5908
www.docboard.org/ia/ia_home
    .htm

Kansas Board of Healing Arts
235 SW Topeka Boulevard
Topeka, KS 66603-3068
785-296-7413
Fax: 785-296-0852
www.ksbha.org

Kentucky Board of Medical
  Licensure
Hurstbourne Office Park
310 Whittington Parkway
Suite 1B
Louisville, KY 40222-4916
502-429-7150
Fax: 502-429-7158
www.state.ky.us/agencies/
  kbml/

Louisiana State Board of
  Medical Examiners
630 Camp Street
New Orleans, LA 70190-0250
504-568-6820
Fax: 504-599-0503
www.lsbme.org

Maine Board of Licensure in
  Medicine
137 State House Station
Augusta, ME 04333-0137
207-287-3601
Fax: 207-287-6590
www.docboard.org/me/me_
  home.htm

Maine Board of Osteopathic
  Licensure
142 State House Station
Augusta, ME 04333-0142
207-287-2480
207-287-3015
www.maine.gov/osteo

Maryland Board of Physicians
4201 Patterson Avenue
Baltimore, MD 21215-0095
410-764-4777
800-492-6836
Fax: 410/358-2252
www.mbp.state.md.us

Massachusetts Board of
  Registration in Medicine
560 Harrison Avenue
Suite G-4
Boston, MA 02118
617-654-9800
800-377-0550
Fax: 617-426-9373
www.massmedboard.org

Michigan Bureau of Health
  Professions
PO Box 30670
Lansing, MI 48909-8170

517-335-0918
Fax: 517-373-2179
www.michigan.gov/
    healthlicense

Minnesota Board of Medical
    Practice
University Park Plaza
2829 University Avenue SE
Suite 500
Minneapolis, MN 55414-3246
612-617-2130
Hearing impaired: 800-627-3529
Fax: 612-617-2166
www.bmp.state.mn.us

Mississippi State Board of
    Medical Licensure
1867 Crane Ridge Drive
Suite 200B
Jackson, MS 39216
601-987-3079
Fax: 601-987-4159
www.msbml.state.ms.us

Missouri State Board of
    Registration for the Healing
    Arts
3605 Missouri Boulevard
PO Box 1335

Jefferson City, MO 65102
573-751-0293
Fax: 573-751-3166
www.pr.mo.gov

Montana Board of Medical
    Examiners
PO Box 200513
Helena, MT 59620-0513
406-841-2300
Fax: 406-841-2363
www.medicalboard.mt.gov

Nebraska Board of Medicine
    and Surgery
Health and Human Services
Regulation and Licensure
Credentialing Division
PO Box 94986
Lincoln, NE 68509-4986
402-471-2118
Fax: 402-471-3577
www.hhs.state.ne.us/reg/reg
    .index.htm

Nevada State Board of Medical
  Examiners
1105 Terminal Way
Suite 301
Reno, NV 89502
775-688-2559
888-890-8210
Fax: 775-688-2321
www.medboard.nv.gov

Nevada State Board of
  Osteopathic Medicine
860 East Flamingo Road
Suite D
Las Vegas, NV 89121
702-732-2147
Fax: 702-732-2079
www.osteo.state.nv.us

New Hampshire Board of
  Medicine
2 Industrial Park Drive
Suite 8
Concord, NH 03301-8520
603-271-1203
Complaints: 800-780-4757
Fax: 603-271-6702
www.nh.gov/medicine

New Jersey State Board of
  Medical Examiners
PO Box 183
Trenton, NJ 08625-0183
609-826-7100
Fax: 609-826-7117
www.state.nj.us/lps/ca/bme/
  bme.htm

New Mexico Medical Board
2055 South Pacheco Street
Building 400
Santa Fe, NM 87505
505-476-7220
Fax: 505-476-7237
www.state.nm.us/nmbme

New Mexico Board of
  Osteopathic Medical
  Examiners
2550 Cerrillos Road
Santa Fe, NM 87504
505-476-4695
Fax: 505-476-4665
www.rld.state.nm.us

New York State Board for
  Medicine/Licensure
State Board for Medicine
State Education Building

Second floor
89 Washington Avenue
Albany, NY 12234
518-474-3817, ext. 560
Fax: 518-486-4846
www.op.nysed.gov

New York State Board for
Professional Medical
Conduct
Department of Health
Office of Professional Medical
Conduct
433 River Street
Suite 303
Troy, NY 12180-2299
800-663-6114
Fax: 518-402-0866
www.health.state.ny.us/
nysdoh//opmc//main.htm
*(Think this Web site address is
long? Just wait until you get
to Washington.)*

North Carolina Medical Board
PO Box 20007
Raleigh, NC 27619-0007
919-326-1100
Fax: 919-326-0036
www.ncmedboard.org

North Dakota State Board of
Medical Examiners
City Center Plaza
418 East Broadway Avenue
Suite 12
Bismarck, ND 58501
701-328-6500
Fax: 701-328-6505
www.ndbomex.com

State Medical Board of Ohio
77 South High Street
17th Floor
Columbus, OH 43215-6127
614-466-3934
800-554-7717
Fax: 614-728-5946
www.med.ohio.gov

Oklahoma State Board of
Medical Licensure and
Supervision
PO Box 18256
Oklahoma City, OK 73118-0256
405-848-6841
800-381-4519
Fax: 405-848-8240
www.okmedicalboard.org

Oklahoma State Board of
 Osteopathic Examiners
4848 North Lincoln Boulevard
Suite 100
Oklahoma City, OK 73105-3335
405-528-8625
Fax: 405-557-0653
www.docboard.org/ok/ok.htm

Oregon Board of Medical
 Examiners
1500 SW First Avenue
Portland, OR 97201-5826
503-229-5770
Fax: 503-229-6543
www.oregon.gov/BME

Pennsylvania State Board of
 Medicine
PO Box 2649
Harrisburg, PA 17105-2649
717-783-1400
Fax: 717-787-7769
www.dos.state.pa.us

Pennsylvania State Board of
 Osteopathic Medicine
PO Box 2649
Harrisburg, PA 17105-2649
717-783-4858

Fax: 717-787-7769
www.dos.state.pa.us

Rhode Island Board of Medical
 Licensure and Discipline
Department of Health
Three Capitol Hill
Providence, RI 02908
401-222-2231
Fax: 401-222-6548
www.health.ri.gov/hsr/blmd

South Carolina Board of
 Medical Examiners
Department of Labor, Licensing
 and Regulation
PO Box 11289
Columbia, SC 29211-1289
803-896-4500
Fax: 803-896-4515
www.llr.state.sc.us/pol/
 medical

South Dakota State Board of
 Medical and Osteopathic
 Examiners
123 South Main Avenue
Suite 100
Sioux Falls, SD 57104
605-367-7781

Fax: 605-367-7786
www.state.sd.us/doh/medical

800-248-4062
www.tsbme.state.tx.us

Tennessee Board of Medical
  Examiners
425 Fifth Avenue North,
1st Floor
Cordell Hull Building
Nashville, TN 37247-1010
615-532-3202
800-788-4123
Fax: 615-253-4484
www2.state.tn.us/health/
  boards/me

Utah Department of Commerce
  Division of Occupational and
  Professional Licensing
Physicians Licensing Board
PO Box 146741
Salt Lake City, UT 84114
801-530-6628
Fax: 801-530-6511
www.dopl.utah.gov

Tennessee Board of Osteopathic
  Examination
425 Fifth Avenue North
1st Floor
Cordell Hull Building
Nashville, TN 37247-1010
615-532-3202
800-778-4125
www2.state.tn.us

Vermont Board of Medical
  Practice
PO Box 70
Burlington, VT 05402-0070
802-657-4220
Fax: 802-657-4227
www.healthyvermonters.info//
  bmp//bmp.shtml

Texas State Board of Medical
  Examiners
PO Box 2018
Austin, TX 78768-2018
512-305-7010

Vermont Board of Osteopathic
Physicians and Surgeons
26 Terrace Street
Drawer 09
Montpelier, VT 05609-1106
802-828-1134
Fax: 802-828-2465
vtprofessionals.org/opr1/
osteopaths

Virginia Board of Medicine
6603 West Broad Street
5th Floor
Richmond, VA 23230-1712
804-662-9900
Fax: 804-662-9943
www.dhp.state.va.us

Washington Medical Quality
Assurance Commission
Department of Health
PO Box 47865
Olympia, WA 98504-7865
360-236-4700
Fax: 360-236-4818
https://fortress.wa.gov/doh/
hpqa1/hps5/Medical/default
.htm

Washington State Board of
Osteopathic Medicine and
Surgery Department of
Health
PO Box 47865
Olympia, WA 98504-7865
360-236-4700
Fax: 360-236-4818
https://fortress.wa.gov/doh/
hpqa1/hps7/Osteopath/
default.htm
*(If you need to take a coffee break in
the middle of typing in these last two
Web site addresses, we understand.)*

West Virginia Board of Medicine
101 Dee Drive
Suite 103
Charleston, WV 25311
304-558-2921
Fax: 304-558-2084
www.wvdhhr.org/wvbom

West Virginia Board of
Osteopathy
334 Penco Road
Weirton, WV 26062
304-723-4638
Fax: 304-723-6723
http://www.wvbdosteo.org

Wisconsin Medical Examining
Board
Department of Regulation and
Licensing
P.O. Box 8935
Madison, WI 53708-8935
608-266-2112
www.drl.state.wi.us

Wyoming Board of Medicine
211 West Nineteenth Street
Colony Building
2nd Floor
Cheyenne, WY 82002
800-438-5784
Fax: 307-778-2069
wyomedboard.state.wy.us

State Boards of Pharmacies

To learn whether a pharmacist is licensed in a particular state or has
had disciplinary actions filed against him or her, contact the board of
pharmacy in that state:

Alabama
10 Inverness Center
Suite 110
Birmingham, AL 35242
205-981-2280
Fax: 205-981-2330
www.albop.com

Alaska
PO Box 110806
Juneau, AK 99811-0806
907-465-2589

Fax: 907-465-2974
www.dced.state.ak.us/occ/
    ppha.htm

Arizona
4425 West Olive Avenue
Suite 140
Glendale, AZ 85302-3844
623-463-2727
Fax: 623-934-0583
www.pharmacy.state.az.us

Arkansas
101 East Capitol
Suite 218
Little Rock, AR 72201
501-682-0190
Fax: 501-682-0195
www.arkansas.gov/asbp

California
1625 North Market Boulevard
Suite N219
Sacramento, CA 95834
916-445-5014
Fax: 916-327-6308
www.pharmacy.ca.gov

Colorado
1560 Broadway
Suite 1310
Denver, CO 80202-5143
303-894-7750
Fax: 303-894-7764
www.dora.state.co.us/pharmacy

Connecticut
165 Capitol Avenue
State Office Building
Room 147
Hartford, CT 06106
860-713-6050

Fax: 860-713-7242
www.ct.gov/dcp

Delaware
Cannon Building
Suite 203
861 Silver Lake Boulevard
Dover, DE 19904
302-744-4526
Fax: 302-739-2711
www.professionallicensing.
    state.de.us

District of Columbia
717 14 Street NW
Suite 600
Washington, DC 20005
877-672-2174
Fax: 202-727-8471
http://hpla.doh.dc.gov/
    weblookup/

Florida
4052 Bald Cypress Way,
    Bin #C04
Tallahassee, FL 32399-3254
850-245-4292
Fax: 850-413-6982
www.doh.state.fl.us/mqa/
    pharmacy

Georgia
237 Coliseum Drive
Macon, GA 31217-3858
478-207-2440
Fax: 478-207-1363
www.sos.state.ga.us/plb/
   pharmacy

Hawaii
PO Box 3469
Honolulu, HI 96801
808-586-2694
Fax: 808-586-2874
www.hawaii.gov/dcca/pvl/
   boards/pharmacy

Idaho
3380 Americana Terrace
Suite 320
Boise, ID 83706
208-334-2356
Fax: 208-334-3536
www.accessidaho.org/bop

Illinois
320 West Washington
3rd Floor
Springfield, IL 62786
217-782-8556
Fax: 217-782-7645
www.idfpr.com/dpr

Indiana
402 West Washington Street
Room W072
Indianapolis, IN 46204-2739
317-234-2067
Fax: 317-233-4236
www.in.gov/pla/bandc/isbp

Iowa
400 SW Eighth Street
Suite E
Des Moines, IA 50309-4688
515-281-5944
Fax: 515-281-4609
www.state.ia.us/ibpe/

Kansas
900 Southwest Jackson Street
Room 560
Topeka, KS 66612-1231
785-296-4056
Fax: 785-296-8420
www.kansas.gov/pharmacy

Kentucky
Spindletop Administration
  Building
Suite 302
2624 Research Park Drive
Lexington, KY 40511
859-246-2820
Fax: 859-246-2823
www.pharmacy.ky.gov

Louisiana
5615 Corporate Boulevard
Suite 8E
Baton Rouge, LA 70808-2537
225-925-6496
Fax: 225-925-6499
www.labp.com

Maine
Department of
  Professional/Financial
  Regulation
35 State House Station
Augusta, ME 04333
207-624-8620
Fax: 207-624-8637
www.state.me.us/pfr/olr

Maryland
4201 Patterson Avenue
Baltimore, MD 21215-2299
410-764-4755
Fax: 410-358-6207
www.dhmh.state.md.us/
  pharmacyboard

Massachusetts
239 Causeway Street
Suite 500
Boston, MA 02114
800-414-0168
Fax: 617-727-2366
www.mass.gov/dpl/boards/
  ph/index.htm

Michigan
611 West Ottawa
1st Floor
PO Box 30670
Lansing, MI 48909-8170
517-335-0918
Fax: 517-373-2179
www.michigan.gov/cis

Minnesota
2829 University Avenue SE
Suite 530
Minneapolis, MN 55414-3251

612-617-2201
Fax: 612-617-2212
www.phcybrd.state.mn.us

Mississippi
204 Key Drive
Suite D
Madison, MS 39110
601-605-5388
Fax: 601-605-9546
www.mbp.state.ms.us

Missouri
PO Box 625
Jefferson City, MO 65102
573-751-0091
Fax: 573-526-3464
www.pr.mo.gov

Montana
PO Box 200513
301 South Park Avenue
4th Floor
Helena, MT 59620-0513
406-841-2356
Fax: 406-841-2343
www.discoveringmontana.com/
    dli/bsd/license/bsd_boards/
    pha_board/board_page.asp

Nebraska
PO Box 94986
Lincoln, NE 68509-4986
402-471-2118
Fax: 402-471-3577
www.hhs.state.ne.us

Nevada
555 Double Eagle Court
Suite 1100
Reno, NV 89521
800-364-2081
775-850-1440
Fax: 775-850-1444
www.state.nv.us/pharmacy

New Hampshire
57 Regional Drive
Concord, NH 03301-8518
603-271-2350
Fax: 603-271-2856
www.state.nh.us/pharmacy

New Jersey
PO Box 45013
Newark, NJ 07101
973-504-6450
Fax: 973-648-3355
www.nj.gov/dps/ca/medical/
    pharmacy.htm

New Mexico
5200 Oakland NE
Suite A
Albuquerque, NM 87113
800-565-9102
505-222-9830
Fax: 505-222-9845
www.state.nm.us/pharmacy

New York
89 Washington Avenue
2nd Floor West
Albany, NY 12234-1000
518-474-3817, X250
Fax: 518-402-5354
www.op.nysed.gov

North Carolina
PO Box 4560
Chapel Hill, NC 27515-4560
919-942-4454
Fax: 919-967-5757
www.ncbop.org

North Dakota
PO Box 1354
Bismarck, ND 58502-1354
701-328-9535
Fax: 701-328-9536
www.nodakpharmacy.com

Ohio
77 South High Street
Room 1702
Columbus, OH 43215-6126
614-466-4143
Fax: 614-752-4836
www.pharmacy.ohio.gov

Oklahoma
4545 Lincoln Boulevard
Suite 112
Oklahoma City, OK 73105-3488
405-521-3815
Fax: 405-521-3758
www.pharmacy.state.ok.us

Oregon
800 NE Oregon Street
Suite 150
Portland, OR 97232
971-673-0001
Fax: 971-673-0002
www.pharmacy.state.or.us

Pennsylvania
PO Box 2649
Harrisburg, PA 17105-2649
717-783-7156
Fax: 717-787-7769

www.dos.state.pa.us/bpoa/
    phabd/mainpage.htm

Rhode Island
Three Capitol Hill
Room 205
Providence, RI 02908-5097
401-222-2837
Fax: 401-222-2158
www.health.state.ri.us/hsr/
    professions/pharmacy.php

South Carolina
Kingstree Building
110 Centerview Drive
Suite 306
Columbia, SC 29210
803-896-4700
Fax: 803-896-4596
www.llr.state.sc.us/pol/
    pharmacy

South Dakota
4305 South Louise Avenue
Suite 104
Sioux Falls, SD 57106
605-362-2737
Fax: 605-362-2738
www.state.sd.us/doh/
    pharmacy

Tennessee
500 James Robertson Parkway
2nd Floor
Davy Crockett Tower
Nashville, TN 37243-1149
615-741-2718
Fax: 615-741-2722
www.state.tn.us/commerce/
    boards/pharmacy

Texas
333 Guadalupe
Tower 3
Suite 600
Box 21
Austin, TX 78701-3942
512-305-8000
Fax: 512-305-8082
www.tsbp.state.tx.us

Utah
PO Box 146741
Salt Lake City, UT 84114-6741
801-530-6179
Fax: 801-530-6511
www.dopl.utah.gov

Vermont
26 Terrace Street
Drawer 09
Montpelier, VT 05609-1106
802-828-2875
Fax: 802-828-2373
vtprofessionals.org/opr1/
   pharmacists

Virginia
6603 West Broad Street
5th Floor
Richmond, VA 23230-1712
804-662-9911
Fax: 804-662-9313
www.dhp.state.va.us

Washington
PO Box 47863
Olympia, WA 98504-7863
360-236-4825
Fax: 360-586-4359
fortress.wa.gov/doh/hpqa1/
   HPS4/Pharmacy/default
   .htm

West Virginia
232 Capitol Street
Charleston, WV 25301
304-558-0558
Fax: 304-558-0572
www.wybop.com

Wisconsin
1400 East Washington
PO Box 8935
Madison, WI 53708-8935
608-266-2811
Fax: 608-267-0644
www.drl.state.wi.us

Wyoming
632 South David Street
Casper, WY 82601
307-234-0294
Fax: 307-234-7226
pharmacyboard.state.wy.us

Acknowledgments

Michael F. Roizen, M.D., and Mehmet C. Oz, M.D.

We were uncertain what to expect when we fielded the initial call from Joint Commission Resources proposing a collaboration. As members of the academic medical community, we are in awe of the Joint Commission, an organization that promotes meaningful improvements in health care delivery. The relationship has been a blessing at many levels, made even more enjoyable by the close friendships we forged with Catherine Hinckley and Eileen Norris. We learned much from our colleagues at the Joint Commission and Joint Commission Resources. We gained new insights into the most important challenges facing American medicine. We gained respect for the magnitude of the patient safety problem and the opportunity to improve it. And we confirmed our belief that we cannot make health care delivery more effective unless we engage our most valuable ally—the patients.

Eileen Norris and Catherine Hinckley from Joint Commission Resources worked tirelessly, and added to their busy schedules our weekly Friday and Sunday conference calls. Joint Commission Resources is lucky to have them. Kelly James-Enger created a treasure trove of information that powered the creation of this book. Our thanks to Joint Commission Resources CEO Karen Timmons for her vision for this project and her willingness to take a risk with our style. That speaks volumes about how much she and her organization care about patient safety. Our thanks, too, to Dr. Dennis O'Leary, president of the Joint Commission, for his insightful leadership and efforts to champion the cause of patient safety.

Ron Geraci's brilliant writing and remarkable editorial insights brought the prose together seamlessly. Gary Hallgren is the most remarkable cartoonist we have ever witnessed. His wit and raw artistic talent yield impressive results. While the hours of conference calls, research, and writing were sometimes exhausting, this powerful team always pulled in the same direction to resolve content and style conflicts. We also owe Ted Spiker a debt of gratitude as he pushed for Ron as our collaborator and provided insights for this work. Finally, our agent Candice Fuhrman's clear vision (and negotiations) allowed this book to grow into the manuscript America deserves.

We also want to thank profusely the group at Free Press (Simon & Schuster) who immediately saw the value of this work and wanted to make our insights part of the American zeitgeist. Thanks especially to our editor Dominick Anfuso, as well as Martha Levin, Jill Siegel, Carisa Hays, Linda Dingler, Beth Maglione, Nancy Inglis, Phil Bashe, and Wylie O'Sullivan.

Thanks, too, to everyone in the Publications Department at Joint Commission Resources, especially Cecily Pew, Johanna Harris, Angela Grayson, Jan Kendrick, Meghan McGreevey, Ilese Smith, Kathy Connors, Shelby Sheehan, Paul Reis, Andrew Bernotas, Rachel Hegarty, and Claudia Appeldorn. And we also extend our gratitude to Hal Bressler, Ken Swezey, Rick Croteau, Ken Hermann, Jan Aleccia, and Laura Shedore for their wisdom and work on the book.

Michael F. Roizen

Anesthesia has always been a leader for patient safety. Jeep Pierce taught me a zealot could change the world, and he did. Bill Hamilton and Jim Arens taught me to ask advice and recruit the best, and Richard Cook, Lyn Kahana, Steve Small, and Paul Barach are the best. They taught me to understand the need for all to make safety a priority. Toby Cosgrove, Joe Hahn, Rob Kay, Mike O'Boyle, and Walt Maurer help make anyone who chooses or refers a patient to the Cleveland Clinic smart. They make safety a part of each person's priorities at the Cleveland Clinic (as Dean Harrison does at Northwestern). I feel fortunate to work with them and with the outstanding clinicians and team in the Anesthesiology, Critical Care Medicine, and Comprehensive Pain Management Division at the Cleveland Clinic—it is no accident that it has been number one in cardiac care as ranked by *U.S. News & World Report* for eleven years in a row.

Special appreciation is due Dr. Walt Maurer, the anesthesiologist at the Cleveland Clinic who chairs the Quality and Safety initiatives, who read and reviewed every chapter. We also need to thank Jennifer L. Roizen and her friends at Caltech who reviewed every edition of each chapter and each cartoon and kept us making each better. And Jeff Roizen pushed to keep every quotation of science pure. I also need to thank Mehmet's family and staff, who accepted phone calls at any hour.

Many colleagues in other specialties at the Clinic provided content and deserve gratitude, especially my administrative associate Beth Grubb, Mary Beth Modic, and other nurses at the Clinic who improved this manuscript, and the RealAge team; the very supportive public affairs group at the Cleveland Clinic, including Jim Blazar, Eileen Sheil, and Mary Claire Burick, taught me to stay on message. And a special thanks to Myrna Pudersen and Joan McGrath and many others who taught me much about how to present ideas.

I need to acknowledge two special people as well: Diane Reverand stated "not to worry about offending medical colleagues—as long as the science was solid, they would understand you were trying to motivate readers to understand they could control their own health and were responsible for doing so and for enjoying the extra energy and vitality"; and the great friend who brought Mehmet and me together—Craig Wynett.

And I need to thank Nancy for her constant love and support. She read this book and used her expertise in critical reading to make our work better. She makes my life better daily.

I hope and believe this book will help YOU to take control of your health experiences and to become a Smart Patient. That would be the best gift any physician could receive.

Mehmet C. Oz

My colleagues at New York Presbyterian–Columbia University have made patient safety part of our institutional culture. I thank our administration, especially Herb Pardes, Steve Corwin, Bob Kelly, Larry Beilis, Ernie Meisner, Deb McGregor, and Laura Forese, for putting these important challenges on my radar screen.

I thank my colleagues in Cardiothoracic Surgery for freeing me to write and brainstorm, especially Eric Rose, Craig Smith, Yoshifuma Naka, Mike Argenziano, Henry Spotnitz, Allan Stewart and the other superb surgeons on our team. The physician assistants, especially Laura Baer, and the nurses in the OR, ICU and floor are the first line of patient safety defense for us. Lidia Nieves, Michelle Washburn, and our über-administrator Diane Amato make sure that no patient (or their medical records) slip through the cracks. Their advice (and scheduling acumen) are priceless.

Thanks to all my colleagues in health care who provided quality control by offering thoughtful feedback on our writing. Thanks to the very supportive public affairs group at New York–Presbyterian, including Bryan Dotson, Alicia Park, and Myrna Manners, who have taught me to stay on message. I appreciate Ivan Kronenfeld for pushing me to speak out.

My parents, Mustafa and Suna Oz, taught me to attack challenges with passion and gusto. My father's attention to detail always made him a safe surgeon; I only hope some of this perfectionist attitude rubbed off on me. My parents-in-law Gerald and Emily Jane Lemole bring wisdom into our family's life daily and are role models to me. They taught me early that the patient is the best guardian of their safety. Finally, thanks to my wife Lisa, who makes my life a continuous blessing-filled journey, and the four particularly loud blessings she bore for me—Daphne, Arabella, Zoe, and Oliver. Thanks for sacrificing numerous weekends to the altar of *The Smart Patient*.

Joint Commission and Joint Commission Resources

This handbook is dedicated to health care organization leaders, physicians, nurses, pharmacists, and other staff at health care organizations in the United States who work daily to heal the sick and injured and who are passionately committed to ensuring the safety of patients and the quality of care provided to them.

We would also like to acknowledge the employees at the Joint Commission on Accreditation of Healthcare Organizations and Joint Commission Resources whose work contributes to the welfare of patients by supporting health care organizations in their quality and safety efforts.

Dennis S. O'Leary
President
Joint Commission on Accreditation of
   Heathcare Organizations

Karen H. Timmons
President
Joint Commission
Resources

Index

About the Authors

Michael F. Roizen, M.D., is a Phi Beta Kappa graduate of Williams College and Alpha Omega Alpha graduate of the University of California, San Francisco, medical school. He performed his residency in internal medicine at Harvard's Beth Israel Hospital and completed a tour of duty in the Public Health Service at the National Institutes of Health in the laboratory of Irv Kopin and Nobel Prize winner Julius Axelrod. He practices and is certified by both the American Board of Internal Medicine and the American Board of Anesthesiology. He is 60 calendar years of age, but lives his RealAge paradigm and has a RealAge of 42.1.

Dr. Roizen is past chair of a Food and Drug Administration advisory committee, has been an editor or associate editor for six medical journals, has published more than 155 peer-reviewed scientific papers, 100 textbook chapters, 30 editorials, and 4 medical books (one a medical best-seller, translated into thirteen languages), and been issued 12 US and many foreign patents. Dr. Roizen is the founder of RealAge, Inc., a San Diego–based company, which includes an interactive Web site located at **www.RealAge.com.** The site addresses health and wellness issues, and the RealAge "Tip of the Day" is subscribed to by over 4.2 million people in North America. Dr. Roizen also developed a program in Partnership medicine first launched at Northwestern Memorial Hospital aimed at helping its members be Smart Patients and reverse biologic aging and live longer, more vibrant lives.

Anesthesiology has led the patient safety movement; Dr. Roizen recruited physicians who are some of the world's safety experts to work in his departments at the University of Chicago and now to the Cleveland Clinic. So when Joint Commission Resources proposed this work, he jumped out of his chair, thrust his fist in the air, and yelled *Yes!*

He has been continually listed since 1989 in the Best Doctors in America reference. He is an avid squash player (captained the U.S. team in what was the forerunner to the Pan American games in 1984) and Cleveland Cavaliers fan. His wife is a developmental pediatrician also listed in the Best Doctors in America. The Roizens have two children, Jenny, a PhD graduate student at Caltech in organic chemistry, and Jeffrey, an M.D./PhD student at Washington University in St. Louis. All three were instrumental in advising on this book. He also has all of Mehmet's numbers on speed dial.

Mehmet C. Oz, M.D., Oz received his undergraduate degree from Harvard University, his MD from the University of organization, has been the nation's leader in continuously improving patient safety and health care quality. The Joint Commission is the principal standards setter and evaluator for a variety of health care organizations, including hospitals, ambulatory care, behavioral health care, home care, laboratories, and long-term care. Joint Commission accreditation is the coveted Gold Seal of Approval and means that a health care organization complies with the most rigorous standards of performance. And that means safe and quality health care for *you*.

Joint Commission Resources (JCR) is the publishing and educational not-for-profit affiliate of the Joint Commission. JCR provides practical, solutions-oriented information on health care quality and medical error prevention to health care organizations around the world. In 2005, the World Health Organization designated the Joint Commission and Joint Commission International (a division of JCR) as a Collaborating Centre on Patient Safety Solutions to identify, develop, and disseminate strategies which will reduce or eliminate the occurrence of errors in health care organizations.

Visit us on the Web at **www.jcaho.org** and **www.jcrinc .com.**

Pennsylvania and an MBA from Wharton School of Business. He was awarded the Captain's Athletic Award for leadership in college and was president of the student body during medical school. In his New York Presbyterian Hospital–Columbia University practice, Dr. Oz has seen success treating patients with a combination of cutting-edge Western techniques like minimally invasive surgery and alternative Eastern therapies such as meditation, massage, and yoga. His research interests include creation of new devices to repair hearts without surgery, heart transplantation surgery, and health care policy. He has authored over 400 original publications, book chapters, abstracts, and books and has received several patents.

In addition to numerous appearances on network morning and evening news programs, Dr. Oz has a series of shows with Oprah teaching America about health and is senior medical adviser to the Discovery Channel, where he has hosted several popular series.

Dr. Oz was elected as a global leader of tomorrow by the World Economic Forum (Davos, Switzerland), was voted the Best and Brightest by *Esquire* magazine and was elected a Doctor of the Year by *Hippocrates* magazine and a Healer of the Millennium by *Healthy Living* magazine. He is annually elected as one of the best physicians in the USA by the Castle Connolly Guide. Dr. Oz lives in New Jersey with his wife and four children.

For more than fifty years, the **Joint Commission on Accreditation of Healthcare Organizations,** a private, not-for-profit